UNDERSTANDING

*L*UMPECTOMY

A TREATMENT GUIDE *for* BREAST CANCER

ROSALIND BENEDET, N.P.
MARK C. ROUNSAVILLE, M.D.

Addicus Books
Omaha, Nebraska

An Addicus Nonfiction Book

ISBN# 1-886039-62-3

Cover design by Peri Poloni
Illustrations by Robert Hogenmiller and Jack Kusler
Typography by Linda Dageforde

This book is not intended to serve as a substitute for a physician. Nor is it the authors' intent to give medical advice contrary to that of an attending physician.

Library of Congress Cataloging-in-Publication Data

Benedet, Rosalind Dolores.
    Understanding lumpectomy : a treatment guide for breast cancer /
Rosalind Benedet, Mark Rounsaville.
        p. cm.
"An Addicus Nonfiction Book."
Includes bibliographical references and index.
    ISBN 1-886039-62-3 (alk. paper)
1. Breast—Cancer—Popular works. 2. Lumpectomy—Popular works. I.
Rounsaville, Mark C. II. Title.

RD667.5.B463 2003
616.99'44906—dc222003018969

Addicus Books, Inc.
P.O. Box 45327
Omaha, Nebraska 68145
www.AddicusBooks.com
Printed in the United States of America
10 9 8 7 6 5 4 3 2 1

Contents

Introduction

As an oncology nurse and a radiation oncologist, we have the privilege of caring for women who have been diagnosed with breast cancer. For more than ten years, we have practiced in the same hospital, where we help women with their journey through breast cancer—from diagnosis to follow-up care.

We acknowledge these women and are grateful to them. Their grace and strength inspire us. They have taught us many lessons. They have shown us that physical and emotional recovery is a process that requires time, effort, information, and open communication. These women have also taught us that the diagnosis of cancer can be used as a powerful motivator for a healthier life, physically and emotionally.

It is our hope that through this book, we may pass on some of the many lessons these women have taught us to help you in your journey through breast cancer surgery.

1

Understanding Breast Cancer

If you're like most women, you've always thought of breast cancer as something that happens to someone else. Until now. If you or a loved one has been diagnosed with breast cancer, you already know the emotional impact of a cancer diagnosis. And you are not alone. Approximately 200,000 American women are diagnosed with breast cancer each year, making it the most common cancer among women.

There is cause for optimism. Breast cancer is one of the most treatable cancers. The survival rate for women with localized, nonmetastatic breast cancer has improved in recent years. The five-year survival rate, which was 72 percent in the 1940s, has increased to 96 percent today. Currently, over 2 million breast cancer survivors live in America.

There are other reasons to be hopeful. Breast cancer treatment has come a long way. Most women no longer have to lose their breast since breast-conserving surgery, or lumpectomy, followed by radiation therapy, has been proven as safe and effective as mastectomy. And the delivery of other treatments, radiation and chemotherapy, has greatly improved. In short, breast cancer treatments are less invasive and easier to tolerate, and physical recovery is faster.

What Is Cancer?

Cancer is a collection of cells that are on a path of uncontrollable growth. Cancer starts when normal cells are damaged, and the genes change, or mutate. Unlike normal cells, which divide a limited number of times before they die, these mutated cells have become "immortal"—they never stop dividing. One cell divides into two, two divide into four, and so on, and this mass of cells forms a *tumor.* This process takes a while. A one-centimeter breast tumor, 3/8th of an inch, and containing about 100 billion cells, takes seven to ten years to form.

Cancer cells have other unique abilities. Individual cells can break off from the main tumor and travel throughout the body by way of our blood vessels and lymph vessels. As a result, tumors may form in distant organs.

Symptoms of Breast Cancer

Breast cancer symptoms may show up in a number of ways. In general, breast cancer causes a change in the breast that is persistent and gets worse over time. Sometimes the change can be detected on a mammogram, sometimes it can be felt, and sometimes it can be seen.

Lump in the Breast

Sometimes breast cancer is found by feeling, or *palpating,* a lump or thickening in the breast or underarm area. It is usually a solitary lump, found in one breast, and it is distinctive—it's usually harder than the surrounding breast tissue. The lump may have been growing for several years before it became large enough for you to notice it. Most of the time it does not hurt, although about 8 percent of the time, there is some pain, discomfort, or a strange feeling associated with the lump.

Although a breast cancer lump typically feels hard, sometimes a cancerous lump can be soft. It is important to know that one cannot tell whether a lump is cancerous simply by touch. Even the most experienced doctor will need to investigate further.

Visible Changes in the Breast

Sometimes breast cancer symptoms are visible. These visible changes persist and generally worsen over time. Some of the visible changes that may indicate breast cancer are:

- Persistent and spontaneous nipple discharge
- A change in the contour of the breast, such as a dimple or a retracted nipple (nipple is pulled inward)
- An enlarged breast that looks red and feels painful and hot (inflammatory breast cancer)
- A persistent sore on the nipple or areola (Paget's disease)

Risk Factors for Breast Cancer

A cancer diagnosis feels like the world as we know it has just fallen apart, but it also bring us deep learning.

—Karen, 46
patient

When a woman is diagnosed with breast cancer, one of her first questions may be, "What could have caused this?" Many women have a sense that something—perhaps something they did—caused the cancer. Please remember that the exact causes of breast cancer are unknown. And most importantly, if you have been diagnosed with breast cancer, don't blame yourself. You are not at fault.

Breast cancer is considered a "multifactorial disease"—many factors interact with each other in ways that we don't yet understand. A few factors are known to increase a woman's risk.

Age

The most significant risk factor for breast cancer is age. Clearly, it is a risk factor that we can do nothing about. As we age, our risk increases for cancer and most other diseases as well. Why? Our *immune systems* weaken as we get older, and we are more susceptible to disease. Approximately 18 percent of women diagnosed with breast cancer are in their forties. About 77 percent of women diagnosed are more than fifty years old.

Childbirth and Menstrual History

Childbirth and menstrual history have a slight impact on a woman's risk for breast cancer. There may be an association between the number of times a woman ovulates during her life and the risk of breast cancer; women who have ovulated more have a higher risk for breast cancer. This would include women who had their first period before age eleven or who never had children. It also includes women who enter menopause later, after age fifty-five; they are at slightly increased risk because they have had more exposure to the hormones estrogen and progesterone.

Pregnancy and nursing decrease a woman's risk of breast cancer. Why? Because breast cells are not fully developed until they lactate, or produce milk. If the breast has fully matured, it is less susceptible to the changes that may promote breast cancer.

Radiation Exposure

High doses of radiation to the chest area, particularly during adolescence, increase the risk of breast cancer. For example, young girls who were treated with radiation therapy for Hodgkin's disease, a cancer of the lymph nodes, have a significant risk as they age. You may be relieved to hear that the radiation from modern mammography probably does not increase the risk of breast cancer. The dose of radiation is very small; mammograms are given infrequently, once or twice a year; and they are started at age forty, when breast tissue is less sensitive to radiation.

Alcohol Consumption

Over the years, studies have suggested that drinking alcoholic beverages increases a woman's risk, but the studies were too small to identify the amount of alcohol that increased risk. Does an occasional drink increase a woman's risk?

In 2002, British researchers analyzed 80 percent of the worldwide studies on alcohol consumption and breast cancer and found that women who consumed alcoholic beverages daily did have an increase in risk. As the number of daily drinks increased, the more the risk increased. Women who consumed more than four drinks a day had a significant increase in risk; women who had only one drink a day had a small increase in risk.

Nutrition and Exercise

To what extent diet affects one's risk for breast cancer is somewhat controversial. Many studies from around the globe disagree. For example, out of twelve studies that examined diet and its association with breast cancer risk, five studies showed an association between a high fat diet and breast cancer; but four studies showed no such association.

Similarly, several studies looked at the role of vitamins in the diet. Two studies found that women who ate foods with the highest amounts of vitamin C and beta-carotene (vitamin A from vegetables) had a decreased risk for breast cancer. A third study found no association with risk.

Is there an association between exercise and risk of breast cancer? Some newer studies suggest that strenuous exercise in one's youth may provide life-long protection against breast cancer. Exercising as an adult may provide additional protection.

Environmental and Household Chemicals

Breast cancer advocacy groups and consumer groups have raised concerns about the possible link between breast cancer and environmental toxins and household chemicals. Laboratory studies offer evidence that such links do exist. On the other hand, current research does not show a clear link between breast cancer risk and pollutants such as DDT, a pesticide, and PCBs, which are used in hundreds of products including paints, plastics, and rubber.

Still, an estimated 85,000 synthetic chemicals are registered for use today in the USA, and more than 90 percent of these chemicals have never been tested for their effect on human health.

Hormone Replacement Therapy

Taking estrogen and progesterone for *hormone replacement therapy* (*HRT*) slightly increases a woman's risk of breast cancer. Only since 2002, when the results of a landmark clinical trial were published, could this statement be made with assurance.

Cancer taught me that life is precious and that I should enjoy each day to the fullest.

—Vivian, 55

The National Institutes of Health initiated the Women's Health Initiative (WHI), a large, well-designed clinical trial to test the risks and benefits of hormone replacement therapy. The WHI study found that during one year's time, among women taking both estrogen and progesterone, 38 out of every 10,000 women developed breast cancer. (These women had been taking HRT for five years.) This compares to 30 women who were taking the placebo.

What about the women who took estrogen alone? After five years, the study found no evidence of an increased risk of breast cancer in women taking estrogen alone.

If you are diagnosed with invasive breast cancer and are taking HRT or estrogen alone, you need to bring this to the attention of your doctor. You'll probably be advised to stop taking hormone supplements, because most breast cancers seem to be stimulated by estrogen and progesterone.

Your doctor may advise you to decrease it gradually to help your body adjust. This regimen works well for many women: Take your usual dose every other day, for one week. Then take your dose every third day for one week. Continue adding a day between doses every week until you are no longer taking HRT. If you wear a patch, cut it in half for one week and then cut that in half for another week.

A final interesting note: Other studies have demonstrated that women who were on HRT when their breast cancer was diagnosed had mortality rates 10 to 15 percent lower than women who were *not* on HRT when diagnosed. Much more research is needed on the risks and benefits of hormone replacement therapy.

Heredity

A small percentage of breast cancers—approximately 10 percent—are related to heredity. How is this determined? In 1994, genetic researcher Dr. Mary-Claire King discovered two genes that she called *BRCA1* and *BRCA2*. Women who carry a mutated form of either of these genes have a 35 to 87 percent risk of developing breast cancer by age 70. These women also have a 17 to 60 percent risk for developing ovarian cancer.

How can you determine whether you have the inherited type of breast cancer? When a family carries the genetic mutation, a pattern emerges—multiple relatives in multiple generations have breast and ovarian cancer. You need to look at your father's side of the family, as well as your mother's. Specifically:

- A number of women (and a few men) over several generations developed breast cancer.
- With each generation, women tended to develop breast cancer at a younger age.
- Some family members had breast cancers in both breasts.
- Since BRCA1 & BRCA2 increase the risk of ovarian, prostate, and colon cancer, some family members also developed these as well.

Certain geographic areas and ethnic groups have a higher incidence of mutated BRCA1 or BRCA2. These include the areas of Iceland and Norway, and individuals of Eastern and Central European Jewish ancestry.

Experts think that about 25 percent of inherited breast cancers are not associated with mutation in BRCA1 or BRCA2. Research is ongoing to identify other genes that may be associated with breast cancer.

Consider Genetic Testing

If you think that you may have the inherited type of breast cancer, you may want to be tested. A commercial blood test has been developed for the presence of mutations in BRCA1 or BRCA2. If you test positive for a defect in BRCA1 or BRCA2, your daughter or other family members may choose to be tested. Remember that not everyone necessarily inherits the gene; each person has a 50 percent chance of inheriting it.

Talk to a Genetics Expert

Genetics counselors are most helpful to a family dealing with inherited breast cancer. These counselors are trained to help individuals decide whether to be tested, and to help them understand the test results. Genetics counselors are trained to help you and your family discuss the emotional issues that often arise, including fear, guilt, anger, and shame.

Genetics counselors can also answer practical questions about the cost of testing and whether insurance pays for it. They are also familiar with the ethical issues regarding patient confidentiality and the legal issues that pertain to a patient's right to health insurance.

2

Getting a Diagnosis

If you have discovered a lump in your breast, or if your doctor has discovered something suspicious in a mammogram, you will need further testing. Of course, this is a stressful time, as you wait and wonder if you have cancer. This stress can be alleviated somewhat with education about what happens next—how breast cancer is ruled out or how it is diagnosed.

Diagnosing breast cancer involves several steps. The first step usually includes an examination by your health care provider. This examination is typically followed by imaging studies, such as a mammogram or an ultrasound or both, then a biopsy of the tissue. This process takes some time, and waiting for appointments and test results can be anxiety producing, to say the least.

Most breast biopsies are negative—no cancer. And the days or weeks that pass before you get a definitive answer will not negatively affect your outcome if you are diagnosed with breast cancer. This period of waiting will not be time enough for the cancer to spread.

Nevertheless, and understandably, most women would like their appointments and results as soon as possible. Generally, you can expedite the process by speaking up. When making appointments, let the office staff know that you are worried and want to be seen as soon as possible. And let your doctors know how you feel and ask their help in expediting the process.

Diagnostic Tests for Breast Cancer

Mammogram

If you discover a breast lump or notice a change in the appearance of your breast, your first step is to have a breast examination by your health provider. If your doctor confirms your finding, the next step is to have a *mammogram*, an X-ray of the breast. A *diagnostic bilateral mammogram* is an X-ray of both breasts.

About 80 to 90 percent of breast cancers can be seen on a mammogram. About half of all breast cancers show up in the X-ray as an irregularly-shaped, solid mass called a "speculated mass." Cancerous tissue is rarely smooth and well-defined. Sometimes these solid masses can be felt by hand, as well.

Find a doctor you can trust, one who will take the time to talk to you.

— Lauren, 37

In about 30 percent of cases, calcium deposits called *calcifications*, which show up in a mammogram, are an indication of cancer. These calcifications are too small to be felt by hand. Their number and pattern tell a physician whether the presence of cancer is likely.

However, it is important to note that not all calcium deposits look suspicious. In fact, *benign* (noncancerous) calcium deposits are a common and normal mammographic finding. Keep in mind that cancer causes calcium deposits; calcium deposits do not cause cancer. So if your calcium deposits turn out to be benign, they do not increase your risk of breast cancer in the future.

How Reliable Are Mammograms?

You've probably heard by now that mammograms are not 100 percent reliable. Some women who have a normal mammogram may have a palpable solid lump or other symptom that may indicate cancer. Breast cancer may not be seen on a mammogram if your breast tissue is dense or thick. The glandular tissue, the part of the breast that makes milk, is dense.

As women age, the glandular tissue shrinks and is replaced by fat. Mammograms are most sensitive after menopause, less sensitive during a woman's forties, and much less helpful in women under age forty. In addition, mammograms are not sensitive in women who are pregnant or breastfeeding.

Certain types of breast cancers are not typically found on mammogram. For example, invasive lobular cancer, inflammatory breast cancer, and Paget's disease usually do not show up on a mammogram.

Breast Ultrasound

An *ultrasound* uses high-frequency sound waves to evaluate a lump. An ultrasound can determine the density of a lump. If it is a fluid-filled cyst, it is benign. If the lump is solid, a biopsy is the next step. Remember that not all solid lumps are cancerous; nevertheless, the tissue must be sampled to know for sure.

Types of Breast Biopsies

The only way to determine with certainty whether a mass in the breast is cancerous is through a *biopsy*. If you have a suspicious finding—something that is seen, palpated, or found on imaging studies—then a biopsy is the next crucial step. During a biopsy, a doctor removes tissue from the suspicious part of the breast. These sample cells are then examined under a microscope by a *pathologist*, a doctor who specializes in examining tissue and diagnosing illness. Any of several biopsy procedures may be used, depending on the nature of the suspicious mass.

Fine Needle Aspiration

A *fine needle aspiration (FNA)* is a biopsy that uses a very fine needle to obtain a sample. Your doctor will use a special needle connected to a syringe. The material drawn into the syringe will be sent to a pathology department. An FNA is less commonly used than a core biopsy.

Core Biopsy

A *core biopsy* is done with a larger needle, which allows a larger tissue sample. If you have a core biopsy, your doctor will administer a local anesthetic and then make a small incision, about one-fourth inch, so that the biopsy needle can be guided easily into your breast. Several tissue samples are extracted through the needle and sent to the pathology department. The procedure is usually painless, although you may feel some pressure as each sample is taken.

Excisional Biopsy

In *excisional biopsy*, performed by a surgeon, the entire suspicious mass is removed. This procedure is performed in an operating room, under local anesthesia. You will be discharged from the hospital the same day. Prescription pain medication is generally needed for just a few days.

Ultrasound-Guided Core Breast Biopsy

Sometimes the area of concern is nonpalpable, or cannot be felt by hand. Your surgeon needs to work with the radiology department to image and localize the area using either a mammogram or an ultrasound. An *ultrasound-guided core breast biopsy* uses an ultrasound to guide the radiologist to position a biopsy needle precisely within the target area. An image-guided biopsy can be either a core or an excision biopsy.

Stereotactic Core Breast Biopsy

A stereotactic breast biopsy is a core biopsy that uses a special mammogram and a computer to position a biopsy needle precisely within the breast to gather a tissue sample. It's the biopsy of choice for calcifications. For this procedure, you will be asked to lie on your belly on a specially designed table and asked to place your breast through an opening in the table. The radiologist administers a local anesthetic and makes a one-fourth-inch incision so the needle can be easily guided into the breast. Using the computer image as a guide, the radiologist takes several tissue samples through the needle. The procedure is painless for most women, although you may feel some vibration or pressure when the samples are taken.

Needle Localization Excision Breast Biopsy

If suspicious tissue cannot be palpated, a needle localization biopsy may be ordered. It is a mammogram-guided excision breast biopsy that removes the entire area of suspicious tissue. This procedure requires that your surgeon collaborate with a radiologist and an X-ray technologist. During this procedure, a wire is inserted though the needle, and a blue dye is injected to color the suspicious tissue. The surgeon is guided by the wire and the blue dye in removing the tissue.

Follow your doctors and nurses orders completely, but always speak up if you have a question, concern, or a fear.

—Carol, 55,
psychologist
breast cancer survivor

Obtaining Your Biopsy Results

When a cancer diagnosis is a possibility, waiting for test results is always difficult. And in fact, it may take a couple of days to get the results of a breast tissue biopsy. In the laboratory, the pathologist must prepare the tissue and put it on small glass slides, which takes twenty-four to thirty-six hours. The pathologist then examines the slides under a microscope and makes a diagnosis; this may take another day. The pathologist then dictates a report, which is sent to your doctor. By the time your doctor receives the final report, it may be five to seven days since the biopsy.

You probably want the results as soon as possible. Speak to your doctor and tell him or her how anxious you feel. Request that he or she call the pathologist for a verbal report, which may be available within forty-eight to seventy-two hours.

Many times this initial pathology report will be very brief, indicating only whether cancer is or is not present. If the biopsy tissue is determined to be cancerous, other tests, such as those to determine how aggressive it is, will be necessary. Sometimes all the needed studies are performed on the biopsy tissue. Other times, these studies are deferred until cancer surgery is performed.

Types of Breast Cancer

Noninvasive Breast Cancers

Lobular Carcinoma in Situ (LCIS)

Lobular carcinoma in situ (*LCIS*) is an abnormal change in some of the cells that line the milk producing lobules in the breast. Many experts do not consider this condition a real cancer, but rather a "marker" that places a woman at a higher risk for developing invasive breast cancer. What are the odds of developing cancer? Out of 100 women with LCIS today, 10 to 15 of them will develop invasive cancer over the next fifteen to twenty years. Half of the invasive cancers will develop in the breast in which the LCIS was found; the other half in the opposite breast.

Given these odds, most experts would not plan surgery. Instead, they would recommend that the woman's doctor monitor her carefully and routinely. Ideally, she would be under the care of a surgeon who is an expert in breast care. Depending on her risk profile, she should be examined two or three times a year and receive yearly mammograms, generally starting at the age of forty. These women, especially, should be taught how to examine their own breasts.

Ductal Carcinoma in Situ (DCIS)

This noninvasive cancer is the earliest stage of breast cancer. *Ductal carcinoma in situ (DCIS)* starts growing within one or more of the milk ducts and remains within the ducts. The term "in situ" means "in place," indicating that the abnormal cells have not invaded surrounding tissue. This cancer does not spread outside the breast, and is considered curable in most every case. The lifetime survival rate is 99 percent.

DCIS is treated by surgical removal. This may be a lumpectomy, possibly followed by radiation therapy, or a simple mastectomy and no follow-up radiation. Extensive DCIS usually affects the entire breast, making mastectomy the better treatment. Because DCIS does not spread outside the breast, removal of lymph nodes is not required and no chemotherapy is required.

Invasive Breast Cancers

Invasive Ductal Carcinoma (IDC)

The most common type of invasive breast cancer occurs in the milk ducts and is called *invasive ductal carcinoma.* It makes up about 80 percent of cases. A diagnosis of this cancer means the abnormal cells have broken out of the ducts and invaded the surrounding breast tissue. A hard lump forms and is typically seen on mammogram.

Treatment for invasive ductal cancer is surgical removal either by a lumpectomy, with radiation therapy or by mastectomy with or without radiation therapy. Since this cancer has the potential to spread, treatment also involves removal and examination of a sentinel node or axillary lymph nodes to determine whether they contain cancer cells. Following surgery, systemic therapy, such as chemotherapy and hormonal therapy, may be recommended to reduce the risk of spreading to other parts of the body. The risk of developing breast cancer in the other breast is about 0.8 percent per year.

Invasive Lobular Carcinoma (ILC)

Ten percent of invasive breast cancers are *invasive lobular carcinoma*, which occurs in the lobes of the breast. Invasive lobular cancers are difficult to detect and are often not seen on mammograms. So when they are discovered, they tend to be larger than invasive ductal cancers.

Women have mistakenly been told that invasive lobular cancer is *bilateral*—that if it occurs in one breast, it will occur in both. In reality, the risk of developing cancer in the other breast is about 1 percent per year, only slightly higher than invasive ductal cancer.

Treatment for invasive lobular cancer is lumpectomy and radiation therapy or mastectomy with or without radiation therapy. Because of the cancer's ability to spread, lymph nodes are also removed and examined. Following surgery, chemotherapy and/or hormonal therapy may be recommended.

Inflammatory Breast Cancer

Inflammatory breast cancer makes up about 1 percent of invasive cancers. It is an aggressive type of cancer that spreads in the breast tissue as well as to the lymph vessels of the skin, causing an inflammation. It's often not found on a mammogram and may not form a lump. However, it has other noticeable symptoms—the breast may feel hot and painful, and look red and swollen. These symptoms can develop quickly over only a few weeks.

Treatment for inflammatory breast cancer starts with chemotherapy followed by typically a mastectomy, and then radiation therapy. Your doctor may then advise hormonal therapy and/or more chemotherapy. In some cases, radiation therapy is given after the initial chemotherapy, and then a lumpectomy.

Other Types of Breast Cancer

Most other types of breast cancer are variations of invasive ductal cancer. *Tubular cancer,* so called because the cells look like little tubes, makes up 1 to 2 percent of cancer cases; it is usually less aggressive. *Medullary carcinoma* (6 percent of cases) can be aggressive or less aggressive. *Mucinous carcinoma* (3 percent of cases) is an infiltrating ductal cancer that makes mucous and has a favorable prognosis. *Papillary carcinoma* (1 to 2 percent) has cells that stick out in finger-like projections and has a favorable prognosis.

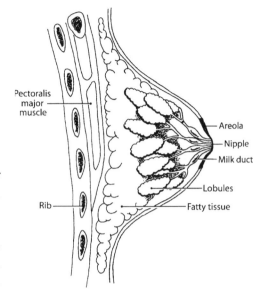

Treatment for these invasive cancers is a lumpectomy with radiation therapy or mastectomy with or without radiation therapy. Lymph node tissue is also sampled. Chemotherapy and/or hormonal treatment may be needed.

Paget's disease (3 percent) forms a lesion on the skin of the nipple and areola, and is highly curable. Treatment for Paget's disease is the surgical removal of the nipple and areola. Axillary lymph node surgery and chemotherapy are not required.

When to See a Breast Specialist

A breast specialist is a surgeon who has interest and experience in matters of breast health and breast cancer. If you have a lump or a visible change, and your doctor says that you are okay and does not suggest follow-up testing, consider a second opinion consultation with a breast specialist. Remember that mammograms are not 100 percent reliable. Even if your mammogram and/or ultrasound are negative, it's wise to see a breast specialist.

A recent study at Northwestern University, published in the journal *Cancer (February 2003)*, emphasizes the importance of a second opinion. According to the study, when women received a second opinion, it resulted in a change in the course of treatment for 20 percent of them. The same study showed that only 46 percent of women had complete treatment options presented to them prior to obtaining a second opinion. Many, who were eligible for lumpectomy, were offered only mastectomy.

Your Treatment Plan

If you are diagnosed with breast cancer, your next step is to meet with a surgeon or breast specialist to discuss the type of surgery that is best for you. You will be able to discuss all your options with your doctors. They will help you understand whether you are a candidate for a lumpectomy, or whether another form of treatment is more appropriate.

3

Your Lumpectomy

In years past, a woman had few choices and not much to say about her breast cancer treatment. The standard treatment was a mastectomy (surgical removal of the breast). These days, a woman has many options and may be asked by her surgeon to decide between a lumpectomy and a mastectomy. Some women are pleased that they have a choice. Other women feel unprepared and insecure about choosing. Many women, however, are still not being given an option.

Over thirty years of research has proven that a lumpectomy is just as safe as a mastectomy in treating invasive breast cancer. Understanding the current approach to the treatment of breast cancer will help you feel confident about making an informed decision. And if you have not been given a choice, this chapter will offer you more information about your options. The better informed you are, the better able you will be to choose doctors who have the training and experience to provide the best clinical and cosmetic outcome.

What Is a Lumpectomy?

A *lumpectomy* is a surgical procedure in which the cancerous tumor is removed from the breast. Lumpectomy is an important advancement in the treatment of breast cancer, because it allows your doctors to treat breast cancer effectively while preserving your breast. Both the appearance and sensation of the breast are usually preserved. This approach is called *breast conservation surgery* (*BCS*). It is a less invasive surgery than mastectomy, so healing time is faster. A lumpectomy may also be referred to as segmental mastectomy, partial mastectomy, or tylectomy.

During a lumpectomy, a rim of healthy tissue around the tumor is also removed. The intent in taking this rim of tissue is to remove any remaining cancer cells. Follow-up radiation therapy to the rest of the breast is routinely advised to kill any remaining cancer cells.

Why Are More Mastectomies Performed?

A physician's training, experience, and bias are the primary reasons fewer lumpectomies are performed. For decades mastectomy was the standard treatment for breast cancer; it is still favored by some physicians and surgeons.

Misconceptions and fear about treatment are other factors. Many women don't have the information they need to make a considered choice. Some women choose to have a mastectomy because they believe it is safer. Other women fear follow-up radiation therapy.

The majority of women diagnosed with breast cancer are eligible for breast conserving surgery but many will have mastectomies instead. Nationwide, 20 to 50 percent of women are having lumpectomies. If you live in the Northeast or on the West Coast, you are twice as likely to have breast conservation surgery than if you live in the Midwest or in the South. In metropolitan areas of the Northeast and the Pacific Coast, breast conserving surgery is much more common than a mastectomy.

Is Lumpectomy Safe?

Although many women are relieved to hear that they will be able to keep their breast, some women worry that breast conservation surgery is not as safe as mastectomy. Many women say that they are willing to sacrifice their breast if it means saving their life; they believe this is the choice they must make. It's important to note that over twenty years of research, involving thousands of women with invasive breast cancer, the survival rate for women having mastectomies is equivalent to that of women having lumpectomies followed by radiation therapy.

> Lumpectomy with radiation therapy is preferable to mastectomy for Stage 1 and State II (up to 5 cm) breast cancers because it provides the same survival rate and preserves the breast.
> —National Institutes of Health 1990 Consensus Conference

The first study to compare mastectomy and breast conservation surgery with radiation therapy was done in Italy during the 1970s. Researchers found no difference in survival rate between the two methods. In the United States, also during the 1970s, the National Surgical Adjuvant Breast and Bowel Project (NSABP) compared lumpectomy alone, lumpectomy and radiation, and mastectomy. This study found similar results: lumpectomy and radiation therapy had the same cure rate as mastectomy.

Scientists have tracked the women who participated in the NSABP study. In 2002, the results of twenty years of follow-up studies made headline news in the United States: for invasive breast cancer, lumpectomy with radiation therapy provides the same survival rate as mastectomy.

Who Is a Candidate for Lumpectomy?

It is estimated that 70 to 90 percent of woman diagnosed with breast cancer are candidates for lumpectomy with radiation therapy. The *ideal* situation is when a tumor is small in relationship to the breast and measures four centimeters or less.

It is also important to have a medical team, skilled in and enthusiastic about breast conservation. You will also need access to a modern radiation therapy department for follow-up treatment.

Will You Also Need Radiation Therapy or Chemotherapy?

As stressed earlier, radiation is almost always recommended after a lumpectomy to destroy any cancer cells remaining in the breast. The purpose of radiation therapy is to prevent *local recurrence*—cancer that could recur locally in the same area of the breast. Studies show that radiation therapy is an important part of breast conservation treatment. The NSABP study showed that after twelve years women who had lumpectomy with radiation had a local recurrence rate of 10 percent. The rate of recurrence with lumpectomy alone was 35 percent. (Those who had mastectomy alone had an 8 percent recurrence rate.)

Are there situations in which a woman might not require radiation therapy after a lumpectomy? A woman who has DCIS with a wide margin (one centimeter) of healthy tissue around her tumor after a lumpectomy, may not require follow-up radiation. However, there is disagreement in the medical community on this matter, and many radiation oncologists recommend radiation therapy for all women who have undergone lumpectomies.

Some women who undergo lumpectomy will also benefit from chemotherapy or hormonal therapy. You and your doctors will make the decision about systemic therapy, based on the nature of your tumor and the cancer's stage, as described in the pathology report, and your overall health.

Chemotherapy and hormonal therapies are called "systemic" treatments because the chemical agents used travel through the body's entire system. The intent is to kill any cancer cells that may have traveled to other parts of the body.

Does Lumpectomy Ever Work for Large Tumors?

In some cases when the tumor is large, breast conservation surgery may still be an option. The most common approach is to start with chemotherapy to shrink the tumor before surgery. Such treatment, prior to surgery, is called *neo-adjuvant* chemotherapy. The chemotherapy is given to shrink a tumor adequately so that a lumpectomy can be performed. The added advantage to this approach is that you and your medical team can tell if your tumor is responding to chemotherapy.

In other situations, a surgeon, who has special training in breast surgery, may be able to perform a lumpectomy and rearrange the remaining breast tissue so that the breast ends up with a nice shape, although smaller in size.

Finally, in cases involving large tumors, after the surgeon performs a lumpectomy, a plastic surgeon may perform a breast reconstruction. This is done by taking a flap of skin, fat, and muscle from your back (*latissimus dorsi muscle*), tunneling it under the skin of your armpit, and creating a breast mound.

If you have a challenging surgical situation and wish to have breast conservation surgery, you may need to talk to several different doctors. You may need a consultation with another surgeon, a medical oncologist, a plastic surgeon, and a radiation oncologist in order to get a full sense of your best treatment plan.

Who Is *Not* a Candidate for Lumpectomy?

Lumpectomy is not always possible. Generally, a lumpectomy is not the appropriate treatment under the following conditions:

- tumor is large in comparison to the size of the breast
- breast has multiple tumors
- presence of inflammatory breast cancer
- presence of extensive DCIS
- a woman has had previous radiation therapy to the chest

A pregnant woman may have a lumpectomy, but radiation therapy must be delayed until after the birth of her baby. The radiation could harm the unborn child.

When Mastectomy Is Better

Some types of cancer involve most of the breast, making a mastectomy the preferred treatment. If you have a large breast tumor, a mastectomy may be the best option.

Mastectomy is also usually recommended for a woman who has multiple tumors in different regions of her breast or if she has been diagnosed with a large, *non-invasive* DCIS, five centimeters or larger. Generally, the only way to adequately remove such a cancer is through removing the breast.

Mastectomy is also the treatment of choice for inflammatory breast cancer, the rare type of cancer in which the breast becomes red, hot, tender, and swollen. This cancer does not form a tumor that can be removed; rather it spreads to the lymphatic vessels in the skin, virtually involving the entire breast. Inflammatory breast cancer is first treated with chemotherapy. After chemotherapy is completed a woman generally undergoes a mastectomy which is followed by radiation therapy.

If a mastectomy is the best treatment for you, breast reconstruction is another option to consider. Reconstruction can be done at the time of the mastectomy or later on, at a time of your choosing. Talk to a plastic surgeon before your mastectomy surgery. If you desire immediate reconstruction, your plastic surgeon and your breast surgeon have to coordinate the surgery.

Preparing for a Lumpectomy

Knowing what to expect during your hospital stay should lessen many of your concerns. Hospital procedures differ. But, most likely, you'll be asked to have routine tests, such as blood pressure, blood test, chest x-ray, and electrocardiogram (EKG) one or two days before your surgery. There are a number of prescription medications, over the counter medications, vitamins, and herbs (such as Aspirin, Advil, Vitamin E, and ginger) that increase bleeding time or may interfere with anesthesia. You'll need to stop taking them a week before surgery. Let your surgeon know all the medications, herbs, and supplements that you are taking.

You'll most likely be asked to fast—not to eat or drink anything after midnight the day before your surgery. You'll probably be admitted to the hospital in the morning and be discharged later on the same day. Sometimes you will be kept overnight and discharged the next morning.

Pack lightly since your stay in the hospital will be a short one. Since all jewelry, including rings and earrings, need to be removed before surgery, it's recommended that you leave them at home. When dressing that morning, think about wearing clothing that will make it easier for you to dress after surgery. Consider a loose fitting blouse, shirt, or dress that buttons in the front. It will be easier for you to put on than a pull-on garment or one that buttons or zips in the back. Or, wear a soft tee shirt or camisole. This will be much more comfortable than a bra after your surgery.

Questions to Ask your Surgeon

- What type of procedure are you recommending?
- How much tissue will be removed?
- Where will the incision be? How large will it be?
- What will my breast look like after the lumpectomy?
- What are the risks and side effects of a lumpectomy?
- What type of anesthesia will I have?
- How long will I be in the hospital?

The Day of Surgery

Your surgery will be performed in an operating room in a hospital or perhaps in a surgery center. As part of the preparation for your operation, you'll be asked to change into a hospital gown. If you wear dentures, a hearing aid, contact lenses, or glasses, they too, will be safely put away and brought to your hospital room after your surgery.

Just before your surgery, an intravenous line (IV) will be put into your arm to provide you with necessary medications and fluids; you may be given medication to help you relax before surgery. You'll be taken to the operating room on a gurney (a bed with wheels) or in a wheelchair; or you may be asked to walk and will be accompanied by a nurse.

Undergoing the Lumpectomy

Once a general anesthesia is given, your surgeon will begin the procedure, first making an incision in the breast. Most surgeons use curved incisions that follow the natural curve of the breast; this allows for better healing.

Then, rather than cut through the tissue, the surgeon will essentially spread the tissue apart until reaching the tumor. The lump and surrounding tissue is cut away and removed along with a rim of tissue around the tumor. The procedure causes little bleeding. The surgeon closes the incision, usually by layers, first breast tissue then fat and skin. Most surgeons use dissolvable sutures that tend to leave less scarring. The incision is covered with a dressing. Once healed, your breast may be smaller and may have a small indentation, but it should retain its original shape.

Axillary Lymph Node Sampling

After the lumpectomy portion of the operation is completed, the surgeon may perform another procedure to remove axillary lymph nodes, located under the *pectoralis muscle* in your armpit. These lymph nodes, along with the breast tissue, will be sent to the pathology department to determine whether the cancer has spread. This procedure is called *axillary lymph node sampling*. The surgeon typically makes a separate incision, about two inches long, in the breast and removes seven to fifteen lymph nodes.

The incision is then closed and a dressing is applied. About half the women who undergo node sampling require a drainage tube in their incisions. Why is a drain needed? It removes blood and lymph fluid that collect as a natural part of the healing process. It also prevents the formation of a pocket of fluid, called a *seroma*, which may develop in the underarm. Whether or not a drain is inserted is based on the surgeon's assessment how much blood and fluid will collect as a result of tissue damage during the operation.

Healing from Axillary Lymph Node Surgery

The axillary lymph nodes are buried deep under the pectoralis muscle, so the procedure results in post-operative pain. After surgery, your arm will be stiff and difficult to move, so that you will need to do arm-stretching exercises. It takes a while for the muscle to heal; complete

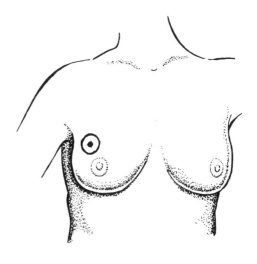

When performing a lumpectomy, the surgeon removes the tumor and a rim of tissue around the tumor with the intention of removing all cancerous cells.

physical recovery takes about six weeks. Often a nerve is severed or damaged, resulting in temporary or permanent numbness in the armpit and in the underside of the arm. After lymph node surgery, there is the lifelong risk of developing swelling in the arm, known as *lymphedema*.

Sentinel Lymph Node Biopsy

Today, a newer, less invasive variation of the lymph node sampling is available called a *sentinel node biopsy*. This procedure samples only the *sentinel node*, which is the first node that drains the area of the tumor. If this node is free of cancer, other nodes need not be removed.

Because sentinel node biopsy is a relatively new procedure, not all surgeons and pathologists are trained and experienced in it. Experts say a surgeon should have done twenty to thirty procedures to become competent at it.

Undergoing a Sentinel Node Biopsy

The sentinel node biopsy is also done under general anesthesia, usually at the time of the lumpectomy. The surgeon injects a small amount of blue dye into the breast; some surgeons use a radioactive tracer instead. The first lymph node (or nodes, sometimes there is a cluster of two or three nodes) the dye or tracer reaches is the sentinel node. The surgeon makes a one-inch incision, removes the node, and hands it over to the pathologist who is standing by in the operating room. The pathologist examines the sentinel node for the presence of cancer cells. If it is negative, then no additional nodes are removed.

If the sentinel node is positive for cancer, the surgeon performs the traditional axillary lymph node sampling. These nodes, as well as all the tissue removed in surgery, will be sent to the pathology department.

A minor side note: the blue dye will make your urine blue for a day or two after the procedure and a small area of your breast may also be blue for several weeks.

Advantages of Sentinel Node Biopsy

Sentinel node biopsy offers a number of advantages over axillary node sampling. It can precisely locate the lymph node that will best indicate the

---

Questions to Ask about Lymph Node Surgery

- Are the lymph nodes in my armpit going to be removed?

- How many lymph nodes will be removed?

- Will I have an axillary or sentinel lymph node biopsy?

- Where will the incision be? How large will it be?

- How will my underarm area look after the node sampling?

- What are the risks and side effects of the node sampling?

- Will I go home from the hospital with a drain in my underarm?

---

spread of cancer. There are fewer complications than with the traditional axillary lymph node surgery. The incision is smaller, about an
inch instead of two inches. Sentinel node biopsy also results in less pain
and discomfort, less potential for a seroma, and less risk of nerve
damage and numbness. Usually a drain is not required after surgery.
Most importantly, there is minimal risk for lymphedema.

After Your Surgery

From the operating room, you'll be taken to a recovery room.
When you awaken, you may be cold, and you will
be covered with a warm blanket. You may feel
cold for a couple of reasons. Operating rooms are
kept cold to prevent the growth of germs. And the
anesthesia sometimes makes you feel cold and can
even cause shivering because if affects the
hypothalamus, the portion of the brain that
controls body temperature.

In the recovery room, a nurse will frequently
check your temperature, pulse, blood pressure,
and your dressing. The nurse will also make sure

> *I recovered well from my
> lumpectomy. At first I thought
> I would need a mastectomy,
> but my doctor explained
> that I was a candidate
> for lumpectomy.*
>
> —Lynn, 40

you are comfortable and will give you medication for pain or nausea, if
needed. You will spend about an hour in the recovery room before
being taken to your hospital room, where you'll be allowed visitors.

Preparing for Discharge from the Hospital

When you're fully awake, usually a couple of hours after being
returned to your hospital room, you'll be encouraged to sit up in bed,
take deep breaths, and cough. This helps clear out your lungs and
prevents pneumonia.

You'll be given clear liquids, like water, apple juice, and tea. Your
IV can be removed when you begin drinking liquids, as long as your
temperature remains normal and the IV is not needed to administer

medications. By early afternoon, most women are ready and eager to go home. Before you're released from the hospital, your nurse will prepare you for discharge. He or she will carefully explain:

- how to care for your dressing
- how to take your pain medication
- when your surgeon wants to see you for a follow-up visit
- how to take care of your drain (if you have one)

Post-Surgical Consultation

About five days after your lumpectomy, you'll have a post-operative appointment with your surgeon. At that appointment your surgeon will check to see how you are healing. Your surgeon will also review your pathology report and begin the discussion about any need for further treatment. If cancer cells were found in the margin of tissue removed from around the tumor, your surgeon may schedule you for a second lumpectomy, called a "re-excision", to remove additional breast tissue. Or, if only a few cancer cells were discovered on the edge of the tumor, your doctors may determine that radiation will destroy any remaining cancer cells.

If follow-up treatment is required, your surgeon will refer you to specialists. A *medical oncologist* will answer your questions about whether chemotherapy or hormonal therapy will benefit you. If you need chemotherapy, it is generally started three to four weeks after your lumpectomy.

You'll be referred to a *radiation oncologist* if radiation therapy is recommended. Radiation therapy usually begins four to eight weeks after a lumpectomy. If both chemotherapy and radiation are recommended, radiation therapy is given after chemotherapy is completed.

4

The Pathology Report

Your lumpectomy is over. Your surgeon has likely given you a preliminary report of how the procedure went. But until the pathology report is ready, the unique characteristics of your tumor will not be known.

After the surgery, all the tissue removed during your lumpectomy is sent to a pathology department for analysis. A *pathologist*, a doctor who specializes in examining tissue and diagnosing disease, will examine the tissue under a microscope and perform a number of tests. Once all the tests are complete, the pathologist will write a comprehensive *pathology report*. Your doctors will use this report to determine the stage of your cancer and recommend the most appropriate treatment.

Tumor Size

After determining the type of cancer present, the pathologist measures the tumor. Since tumors are oddly shaped, the pathologist records the largest diameter seen on the pathology slide. The results are reported in centimeters (cm). An inch is about 2.5 centimeters.

Tumor Margins

Important to the pathologist's role is determining whether the tumor was completely removed. Cancer is often shaped like a crab, and a surgeon may see the body of the crab, but not the microscopic "claws" that may extend into surrounding tissue. Surgeons must rely on a pathologist to tell them if the cancer was completely removed. If it appears that the entire cancer has been removed, the margin—the rim of tissue around the tumor—is called *negative* or *uninvolved*. When cancer cells appear at the edge of the excised tissue, the margins are called *positive* or *involved*.

The pathologist also measures the thickness of the margins. What is considered an adequate margin? Answering this important question is a collaborative effort among your surgeon, your radiation oncologist, and the pathologist.

Ask your doctor or nurse to explain your pathology report to you. Don't be intimidated by those medical terms—- you will be able to understand it.

—Rosalind
oncology nurse

Lymph Node Status

If lymph node surgery was performed, the pathologist counts the number of lymph nodes that were removed and examines them for the absence or presence of cancer cells. Lymph node status is an important predictor of metastatic disease. The more lymph nodes that test positive for cancer, the more likely that the cancer has spread beyond the breasts.

Mitotic Index

If the cancer is invasive, the pathologist counts the number of cells that are in the process of dividing. Less aggressive cancers tend to have fewer dividing cells. The most aggressive cancers have many dividing cells because they are growing rapidly. Cell division is called *mitosis*, so this is called the *mitotic index*.

Vascular and Lymphatic Invasion

If the cancer is invasive, the pathologist will also check for cancer cells in the middle of blood or lymphatic vessels. The pathology report will state whether vascular or lymphatic invasion is present or absent. If vascular or lymphatic invasion is present, the cancer cells are more likely to spread to the underarm lymph nodes and beyond.

DNA Analysis

Cytometry is a way of measuring the amount and type of DNA in invasive cancer cells. DNA is the genetic material found in the nucleus of each cell. Cancer cells that contain the normal amount of DNA are called *diploid*. Cancers that have too much or too little DNA are termed *aneuploid*. Aneuploid cancers are more likely to spread into the bloodstream.

S-Phase

Cytometry is also a way of measuring the percentage of invasive cells duplicating their genetic material in preparation to divide. The period immediately before a cell divides is called the S-phase (*synthetic*). The percentage of cells in the S-phase tells how fast a cancer is growing or diving. Cancers with an S-phase of over 10 percent have more of a chance of spreading into the blood stream.

Her2 Test

The human epidermal growth factor receptor 2, known as *Her2*, is a protein receptor found on cells and is a key component in regulating cell growth. When the Her2 gene is altered, extra Her2 may be produced. About one-fourth of invasive breast cancers have an overexpression of Her2. Knowing the Her2 receptor status of invasive cancer is important because Her2-positive tumors tend to be more aggressive.

Hormone Receptor Test

Normal breast cells have receptors that make them sensitive to the female hormones estrogen and progesterone. Invasive breast cancer cells may or may not retain their receptors, depending upon the degree of mutation that has occurred. Estrogen and progesterone reception is a powerful predictor of the response to hormonal treatment.

Grading Invasive Breast Cancer

Grading, which should not be confused with staging, is a system for reporting how aggressive cancer cells are. Grading involves comparing the appearance of the cancer cells with normal cells. Well-differentiated cancers look more like normal cells and are slower growing. Poorly-differentiated cells, which are more chaotic and do not resemble normal cells, are faster growing. Moderately-differentiated cells are in between.

The Bloom-Richardson Grading System is the most commonly used system to grade invasive cancer in the United States. It grades the degree of malignancy and is used to predict the chance that cancer cells will spread into the bloodstream.

Grade I: Low degree of malignancy
Grade II: Intermediate degree of malignancy
Grade III: High degree of malignancy

This grading system is based on the appearance of the cancer cells, the appearance of the nucleus within each cancer cell, and how quickly the cells are dividing.

Staging Breast Cancer

One of the most important questions is whether the cancer has left the breast and spread to other organs. A woman's *prognosis*, the projection of disease-free survival, is based on the stage of the cancer.

Staging is a process that requires careful analysis of the type and size of the tumor, lymph node involvement, and perhaps other tests to look for cancer in other parts of the body. The surgeon starts the process by making a clinical estimate based on what he or she feels and sees during surgery. Later, the pathologist confirms the surgical findings microscopically and performs a number of tests on the tissue. Last, the medical oncologist may order such tests as a bone scan or CT scan (computer tomography) to look for cancer in other parts of the body.

Breast Cancer Stages

Stage 0

Ductal carcinoma in situ (DCIS) or lobular carcinoma in situ (LCIS) of any size. (Lymph nodes are not sampled.)

Stage I

An invasive tumor that measures 2 centimeters or smaller in diameter, and has not spread to the lymph nodes in the underarm area. (2.5 cm equals 1 inch.)

Stage II

An invasive tumor that measures between 2 and 5 centimeters in diameter and/or has spread to the lymph nodes under the arm.

Stage IIIA

An invasive tumor that measures larger than 5 centimeters in diameter and/or has spread to underarm lymph nodes, causing them to adhere to one another or the surrounding tissue.

Stage IIIB

An invasive breast cancer of any size that has spread to the skin, chest wall, or supraclavicular or internal mammary lymph nodes (located beneath the breast and inside the chest).

Stage IV

An invasive cancer of any size that has spread to distant sites such as bones, liver, or lungs, or to lymph nodes not near the breast. Cancer that has spread to distant sites is said to have *metastasized.*

Don't be shy about seeking a second opinion and select your team of physicians wisely.

— Rose, 59

Although staging is important, you must remember that you are an individual, not a statistic. Recovery is a complex, sometimes mysterious, process. It includes the unique characteristics of your tumor and how you, as a unique individual, respond to treatment.

Consider a Second Opinion Pathology Review

Since appropriate treatment starts with and depends on an accurate pathology report, you may want to consider having a second opinion pathology review. This means that another pathologist, preferably at another hospital, examines your pathology slides under a microscope. A second opinion may find a tumor to be smaller or larger than originally thought. Or a cancer may be found to be less or more aggressive than originally reported.

Consider a second opinion if your pathology report is incomplete and does not cover all the categories mentioned in this chapter. Consider a second opinion if the report is inconsistent. For example, a report that says a tumor is well-differentiated (slow growing) but has a high S-phase (fast growing) is inconsistent and calls for reexamination.

Grading DCIS

If you have been diagnosed with DCIS, the early-stage noninvasive cancer that appears in milk ducts, a second opinion pathology review is particularly important. DCIS is graded differently from invasive cancers, and can be more difficult to diagnose. Sometimes it is mistaken for a low-grade invasive ductal cancer. Conversely, benign noncancerous changes are sometimes mistakenly diagnosed as DCIS.

To predict the rate of local recurrence, the Van Nuys Prognostic Index (VNPI) has been developed. It is a scoring system that is based on cell type, size of the DCIS tumor, and size of the healthy rim of tissue that surrounds the DCIS tumor. The VNPI will help your doctor determine if your lumpectomy is all the treatment that you need. If the VNPI is high, your doctor may recommend more treatment, such as more surgery to remove a wider rim of healthy tissue, radiation therapy, and/or hormonal treatment.

5

Recovering at Home

You'll probably be surprised at how well you'll feel after your lumpectomy. Still, you'll need to take it easy for awhile. You may have the help of friends and relatives, but you'll probably find that most of your care will be up to you. Here are some suggestions to help you during the first few days that you're home.

Energy and Bed Rest

Although you probably won't have a great deal of postsurgical discomfort, you'll probably feel tired both from the surgery and from the medications you received. In fact, by the time you arrive home, your first impulse may be to go to bed and stay there until you feel more energetic. Taking a nap is fine. But bed rest is not encouraged, because inactivity leads to more fatigue.

How much can you do, and how soon? Follow the guidelines from your doctor but a good rule of thumb is to do what you feel capable of doing.

You can resume your normal, daily activities such as grooming, bathing, dressing, and eating, without assistance. However, for more strenuous household tasks, you will need the help of family and friends. Avoid any heavy lifting, pushing, or pulling for six weeks. You may do light household activities such as washing a few dishes, making a simple meal, and setting the table. Be gentle in using your affected arm. There's a natural tendency to favor the side where the operation was done and to hold your arm stiffly at your side. Try to keep your affected arm, neck, and shoulder relaxed.

Managing Pain

You may feel some pain at the surgical site in the breast and/or in the underarm area. If you do, there are a number of steps you can take to ease the pain.

Prescription Pain Medication

If your doctor has given you a prescription for a pain medication, be sure to have the prescription filled right away and take the prescribed dose as recommended on a regular schedule. Some women resist taking these medications because they worry about dependency. But in all likelihood, you won't need to take a prescription medication for more than a few days and nights, so dependency is not really an issue.

Give yourself permission to slow down and get extra rest.

—Patricia Ann, 57

Take your pain medication regularly, before pain intensifies. If you wait until the pain starts, you'll have to endure the discomfort until the medication begins to work. And you will probably take more medication in the long run.

Over-the-Counter Medications

Side effects of prescription drugs, especially sleepiness and constipation, bother some women. These side effects are rarely if ever a problem with over-the-counter (OTC) pain relievers, such as acetaminophen (Tylenol). Try taking an OTC pain reliever on a regular schedule; you may be able to cut back on the prescribed pain medication. Keep your doctor informed about what OTC medications you are taking. And be sure to avoid OTC products that contain aspirin

41

like (Anacin) or ibuprofen (Advil). Both aspirin and ibuprofen have a blood-thinning effect that inhibits clotting.

Cold Packs and Heat Packs

If you had lymph nodes removed, your greatest discomfort is usually in the underarm area. Cold packs, and later warm packs, may help relieve the discomfort. An ice treatment is best right after surgery.

You can purchase soft gel packs (the kind athletes use) at a pharmacy and keep them in the freezer until you're ready to use them. A bag of frozen peas or frozen cranberries works just as well. Wrap the cold bag in a soft cotton towel so that it doesn't come into direct contact with your skin. If this treatment helps, you can leave the ice pack in place for as long as twenty minutes. Then, remove the pack for ten minutes before applying it again.

Heat may be comforting, but you must wait at least seven days after surgery before using a heating pad, because it can increase post-surgical swelling. The area around your incisions will be numb and less sensitive to heat, so be careful not to burn yourself with a heating pad. Use only a low to moderate heat setting.

Caring for Your Dressing

You'll have a dressing that needs to stay in place for two to five days or until your follow-up visit with your surgeon. Your hospital nurse will tell you what your surgeon prefers. You may have a simple gauze dressing or an elastic dressing that covers your entire torso.

Keeping the dressing dry is essential. If the dressing becomes wet, the incision won't heal properly, and the risk of infection increases. You might choose to take a sponge bath or you may sit in a shallow bath, but postpone taking a shower until the dressing is permanently removed.

Caring for Your Drain

Drains may be inconvenient and unattractive, but they serve a necessary function. If you have a drain, you'll go home with it. Your hospital nurse will review instructions for emptying it before you leave the hospital. Each day, the amount of drainage should decrease. The color of the fluid will change over the next several days, from red to light pink.

If you notice there is no drainage, you may have a blocked drain. The following "milking" technique may open it. Pinch off the end of the drain nearest your body with your left hand. With wet gauze in your right hand, pinch just under your left hand, and squeeze a few inches down the tube. While still holding the tube with the right hand, release the left, move it down behind the

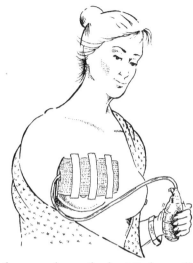

Before you leave the hospital, you'll be instructed on how to empty your drain, which will collect blood and fluids that normally collect at the incision site.

right hand, and pinch the tube again. Resume the milking action with your right hand, pinching off with your left hand each time so the suction action pulls any blockage down the tube. If this technique doesn't work, and you're still not getting drainage, call your surgeon.

If you notice that your drainage is increasing rather than decreasing, you are probably overusing your affected arm. Use that arm more gently, and notice if there is less drainage the next day. If the drainage continues to increase, call your surgeon.

Meals at Home

Keeping good nutrition in mind, you may eat foods that appeal to you when you first arrive home. It's important to drink plenty of water and other hydrating liquids—they help the body's cells do their work. Non-caffeinated drinks are recommended because caffeine is dehydrating.

Managing Constipation

Constipation may result from general anesthesia and pain medications. Here are some specific recommendations to help with constipation:

- Drink ten glasses of hydrating liquids a day.
- Increase the fiber in your diet with fruits, vegetables, and whole grains.
- As you resume exercise, pay special attention to walking, which stimulates the movement in your colon that brings on a bowel movement.
- Eat at least five prunes a day or drink a daily glass of prune juice. Prunes have a nutritional component that gives them a well-deserved reputation for promoting bowel movements.

If the above suggestions don't ease constipation, ask your doctor to recommend an over-the-counter aid. The following are effective, yet mild on the digestive track: a stool softener such as Colace, a fiber supplement such as Metamucil, or a medication that brings on a bowel movement such as Senecot.

Sleeping at Night

Sleeping well is essential for physical and emotional stamina. However, you may find falling asleep and staying asleep a challenge in the weeks after surgery. You will likely be more comfortable if you position several pillows around yourself. Place several large pillows behind your back. Use more pillows to raise the arm on your affected side. Your arm should be higher than your heart when you're leaning back comfortably against the pillows. This will also help minimize post-surgical swelling.

The following guidelines will also help you get the best rest possible:

- If you are taking pain medication, take a pill forty-five minutes before you go to bed.
- Eat a sleep-promoting snack. Foods that contain the amino acid tryptophan help promote sleep, but you need to eat them at least an hour before you go to bed. These foods include cottage cheese, yogurt, turkey, fish, and bananas.
- Avoid "wake-up" foods that may cause indigestion. These include spicy foods, alcohol, citrus juice, carbonated or caffeinated beverages, chocolate, peppermint, fatty or greasy foods, and whole milk dairy products.
- Avoid drinking fluids within four hours of your bedtime (avoid waking up to go to the bathroom).
- Keep your bedroom dark, quiet, and cool. The atmosphere of your bedroom should be calm and relaxing.
- Establish a pleasurable and relaxing sleep ritual. Each night before you fall asleep, listen to soothing music, read a relaxing book, or say prayers.
- Establish a sleep routine. Go to bed at the same time every night. Set your alarm clock so that you wake up the same time each morning, then get up with the alarm—even if you are tired. If you need a nap later in the day, make sure that you nap for no longer than one hour. Napping longer than that is likely to interfere with your night's sleep.
- If you wake up during the night, avoid turning on bright lights as this will wake you up. Instead leave a night light on so that if you need to go to the bathroom you can find your way. To help yourself fall asleep again, repeat your relaxing sleep ritual.

- If hot flashes wake you up, sleep in a cold room, under light covers, in a light, sleeveless nightgown and no socks.
- If you are experiencing sleep problems because of anxiety, try writing down your concerns in a journal or jotting down questions that you need to ask your doctors.

Finally, if you are following these recommendations and still having trouble falling asleep or staying asleep, speak to your doctor. He or she may prescribe a medication that can help you sleep. If your depression and anxiety deepen, ask your doctor to refer you to a caring mental health professional. Sometimes talking about concerns can ease anxiety and depression. Remember, sleeping well is essential to your recovery.

Your First Post-Operative Visit

At your first follow-up visit to the surgeon, usually five days after surgery, your doctor will check your incisions and see how you are healing. If you have a drain in place, your doctor will probably remove it.

Surgeons use different kinds of stitches, and some of them don't have to be removed at all. Absorbable stitches, as the name implies, dissolve on their own. The steri-strips (a special kind of tape) that are placed over absorbable stitches usually remain in place for about seven to ten days, so your surgeon won't remove them during this visit. The strips will fall off on their own.

Your pathology report will probably be ready, and if your lymph nodes were sampled, those results will likely be ready, as well. Your surgeon will review those results with you, discuss additional treatment, if appropriate, and refer you to a medical oncologist and/or a radiation oncologist.

You may want to have a family member or friend accompany you to this important appointment. The doctor will have many things to explain, and you may have questions, as well. Many women find it very helpful to have someone else there to help listen and remember the details.

Looking at Your Incision

Although you may feel relieved that you have kept your breast, you may also feel sad and disappointed over the change in the appearance of your breast. A scar on any part of your body can be upsetting, and it is understandable that you may be particularly concerned with scars on your breast. Remember, in time scars fade and slight depressions fill in.

Your first post-operative visit may be the first time you're able to look at your incision. Many women find this difficult to do. If you are having difficulty looking at yourself in the mirror, try looking down at your incisions. Gradually you'll become more comfortable with the changes in your breast.

I have learned that in order for me to give of myself to others, I need to take care of myself.

—Paula, 42

Early on, your arm, underarm, and breast may be swollen from the surgery. Post-operative swelling is temporary, and it's a normal part of healing. After about six weeks, the swelling lessens.

You may also notice bruising in the breast and underarm area. This, too, is normal, and will also disappear in about six weeks. The bruise marks will gradually change color, from a dark blue to purple to a light yellow. If you had a sentinel node biopsy, an area in your breast may have a blue stain; this, too, fades in time.

As your incisions heal, a scar will form; it will be dark pink at first, but will fade to light pink. Over time (sometimes as long as a year), the scar will continue to fade and take on the color of your skin. When you run your finger over the scar, you will feel a firm ridge, called a healing ridge, that softens as healing progresses.

While the scars are healing, they may itch. You can help relieve the itching by massaging a mild, unscented lotion into the skin.

Caring for Your Incision

It is important to look at your incision daily for signs of infection: increased redness, swelling, warmth, pain, and drainage around the incision. If you notice any signs of infection, call your surgeon's office. If you notice a soaking stain on your dressing or undergarments call your surgeon's office. Tell the medical staff the size and color of the drainage (such as the size of a quarter or a grapefruit). A red stain indicates bleeding; a greenish stain indicates infection. Normal drainage is yellowish pink or brown.

Wash your incisions with mild soap and water to help reduce the risk of infection. Don't be afraid to touch them. Since the area will be numb, it may feel unusual. You can use a washcloth if you prefer, but no harsh scrubbing. After you wash, pat the areas until they are completely dry. Always use a fresh, clean towel to reduce the risk of infection.

Don't submerge your torso in water until your surgeon gives you the okay. After the drain has been removed, you can take a shower the next morning.

Possible Incision Complications

Although an infection at the site of the incision is unlikely, be alert to signs of infection. As mentioned earlier, sometimes a pocket of fluid, called a seroma, develops in the armpit. If this occurs, you will feel the bulge when you rub your arm against your body. A seroma may feel uncomfortably large. Although it usually shrinks by itself in about six weeks, you and your surgeon may decide that you will be more comfortable if it's drained. The quick procedure is done in the doctor's office. With little if any pain, a very small needle is inserted into the seroma, and the fluid is removed.

Noting Sensory Changes

As you touch your incisions and scars, your affected breast and underarm, you may discover that some areas lack sensation and others are extremely sensitive to touch. Over the next year or so, you will probably experience ever-changing sensations. You may feel sharp pain or a dull aching, heaviness, stiffness, burning, or a "pins and needles" sensation in your affected breast, armpit, and arm on the side of your surgery. These sensations may increase when you're tired or feeling stressed. Changes in the weather can also make a difference.

If lymph nodes were removed, additional nerves may have been severed or stretched. As a result, you may feel some numbness in your armpit and on the back of your arm. In time, you may regain some or all of the feeling in these areas.

Minimizing Swelling

In the days immediately after your surgery, you can minimize swelling in your arm and breast by following these guidelines:

- Don't overuse your arm. Gentle, normal movements are fine, but this is no time to be lifting boxes or spending a lot of time at the keyboard.
- When sitting or lying, rest your arm comfortably on several pillows so that your hand and forearm are higher than your heart.
- Perform the arm pumps described in the exercising chapter, once or twice a day, starting the day after surgery.

Choosing Comfortable Undergarments

During the first few weeks after a lumpectomy you may find your undergarments uncomfortable. After your dressing has been removed, a loose undershirt or camisole will probably be more comfortable next to your skin than your regular bra. The most comfortable fabric next to your skin is cotton or silk. You will probably want to wear cotton right after surgery since it is easy to wash. Silk is best to use after your incision has healed completely. Silk is especially comfortable if your skin is extra sensitive to touch.

You may find that a garment with some elasticity that exerts pressure on the lumpectomy side feels comforting and offers some support. You may find that a sports bra feels good because it exerts some pressure. If a sports bra exerts too much pressure, try a cotton camisole with some Lycra. Try them with and without a built-in bra, depending on how much support you need.

Try on your bras to see if they are comfortable. If they are comfortable with the exception of a part of fabric that rubs the incision, cut out the section where it rubs. If you can't make your bras work and you are more comfortable wearing a bra, try a *post-surgery bra*, designed to be worn after breast surgery. They may be found in the lingerie section of large department stores and in stores that specialize in home health care products.

Driving

You can begin driving again when you feel ready, as long as you are no longer taking narcotic pain medication. If the cross-strap of your seatbelt is uncomfortable, slip a small pillow between the belt and your chest.

At first, it may feel uncomfortable to turn the wheel, especially when you're parallel parking. This movement will not harm or reopen your incisions.

Going Back to Work

Weigh your readiness to return to work against your progress in healing. Is your job physically or emotionally demanding? Discuss your working conditions with your surgeon. Of course, any further treatment you may require will also influence your return to work.

Once you are back at work, should you tell your co-workers that you have had breast surgery? Some women prefer to keep the matter private. On the other hand, if no one knows, they can't offer you support. You need to do what feels right for you. If you join a support group where some members have already gone back to work, you can learn from some of their experiences.

As for legal rights, under the Federal Rehabilitation Act of 1973, federal employers or companies receiving federal funding cannot discriminate against cancer survivors. But state laws vary, and how protection laws apply in the private sector varies.

6

Your Exercise Program

When we think of recuperating from surgery, we may think of getting cozy in bed, eating treats, and watching television. These activities can play a part in your recovery. But exercising—walking, stretching and light weightlifting—will speed your recovery and help you regain your energy, flexibility, and strength. In fact, if you feel like it, take a short walk on your first day home from the hospital.

On your second day home from the hospital, you may begin gently stretching your neck, shoulders, and arms. In about three weeks, you may begin some light weightlifting exercises. It is important to start slowly and gradually increase the pace and intensity of exercising.

A Daily Walk

Walking every day, preferably in nature, will not only make you feel more energetic, it also will help your emotional and physical recovery. In fact, research has shown that a daily walk increases energy levels and helps elevate one's mood. It's often recommended as a treatment for mild to moderate depression.

The goal is at least a daily thirty-minute walk, but you don't have to walk the full thirty minutes your first day out. You might want to start with one or two five-minute walks every day, then gradually lengthen your walking time. If it's impractical to spend half an hour walking, try for three ten-minute walks daily. As you increase the duration of your walks, increase the pace as well.

The most beneficial kind of walking is continuous. Stop-and-go activities—running errands, housework, even gardening—are likely to make you more tired, whereas continuous walking actually makes you feel more energetic.

Keep in mind that if you undergo any additional treatment, such as chemotherapy or radiation therapy, a daily 30-minute walk is also recommended; walking improves energy and may help offset the side effect of fatigue.

Importance of Stretching

You may notice that your underarm feels tight, and you may feel like there is a tight band running down the inside of your arm. Regular stretching is essential to achieve flexibility. These stretches will feel uncomfortable, but should not be unbearable. Scar tissue is not elastic, and you're pulling on it when you stretch; this explains the discomfort. But that pulling sensation is an indication that you are making progress. As you continue to stretch every day, you will gradually regain your flexibility and begin to feel more comfortable.

The following guidelines apply to all stretching exercises:

- Stretch once or twice a day, starting the second day that you're home from the hospital.

Benefits of a Daily Walk

- Improves energy
- Helps mental functioning
- Improves bone density, reducing the risk of osteoporosis
- Exercises your heart and lungs, reducing your risk of heart disease
- Improves your mood
- Reduces stress
- Helps you sleep better at night
- Reduces the number and intensity of hot flashes and night sweats
- Regularizes bowel movements
- Helps with weight loss
- Reduces the risk of lymphedema
- Enhances your immune system

- Each time you stretch, try to reach a little bit farther than you did before. Stop and hold the stretch as soon as you feel your incision pulling.
- Hold the stretch for at least fifteen seconds. Do not bounce when stretching.
- Remember to breathe before, during, and after each stretch.

Before You Exercise

Get Comfortable

Use your exercise session as a time to relax. Keep the room quiet and dimly lit. The room temperature should be moderate. If you're doing floor exercises, it's advisable to use a carpet, rug, or exercise mat. The best clothing is loose and comfortable, such as sweat pants with an elastic waist band. Always remove your shoes.

Get Relaxed

It's helpful to do the relaxation exercises before and after your exercise routine. When you are completely relaxed, your respiration slows, your blood pressure falls, and your heart rate decreases. Do these exercises anytime you want to calm yourself and feel more relaxed. Try these exercises at bedtime to help you fall asleep, or during your radiation or chemotherapy treatments.

Two simple relaxation exercises are extended exhalations and an imagery exercise called favorite place. After doing these two exercises, you are likely to feel calm, relaxed and more refreshed than before, as if you had taken a long rest.

Extended Exhalations

Lie down or sit in a comfortable chair. Close your eyes and focus all your attention on your breathing. Inhale and exhale slowly and deeply for at least three long breaths. Inhale through your nose. Exhale through your mouth.

Continue focusing on your breathing, making your exhalations *longer* than your inhalations. Then try closing your mouth and exhaling through your nose. While maintaining the slow, steady, deep rhythm of breathing, continue to inhale and exhale, making your exhalations longer than your inhalations.

As you settle into a steady breathing pattern, you may find that your mind wanders. If so, shift your focus back to your breath. Some women like to think of healing words, focusing on a word or phrase like " hope," "love," or "healing energy." Try to spend a little more time on this relaxation exercise each time you do it.

Favorite Place

Lie down or sit in a comfortable chair. Close your eyes. First, focus on your breathing, practicing the extended exhalations for a few breaths. Then think of a time when you felt relaxed and peaceful—perhaps during a walk in the park, a day at the beach, or sitting on your porch. Focus intently on the sights, smells, and physical sensations associated with that event. Focus on this image for at least five minutes. Try to spend a little more time on this relaxation exercise each time you do it.

Shoulder Shrugs

You may notice that your neck and shoulder feel tight, stiff, and sore on the side of your surgery. For relief, try several shoulder shrugs.

You may begin this simple stretch the day after you return home. Since your arms remain at your sides, this stretch can be done easily even if you have a drain. Do shoulder shrugs at least once every day, or before you begin doing other stretches and exercises.

Position: Stand with your arms by your sides.

Motion: Raise your shoulders toward your ears, hold for a few seconds, and then lower them and relax your shoulder and neck.

Repetitions: 3

Arm Pumps

After surgery, you may notice that your upper arm is swollen. Any time you notice swelling in your hand or arm, it indicates a buildup of lymphatic fluid. Arm pumps increase lymphatic drainage, reducing the swelling.

Start the arm pump exercise the day after surgery. Arm pumps can be done even while the drains are still in place. Repeat the exercise at least once every day, or any time you notice swelling in your hand or arm. Be sure to let your surgeon know about the swelling.

Position: Seated, with your affected arm, palm up, resting on pillows so it's positioned higher than your heart. (For increased comfort, you might also want a pillow supporting the small of your back.)

Motion: While making a fist, bring your hand toward your shoulder. Make a hard fist, squeezing hard and holding it for a few seconds. Then make a hard muscle in your biceps. Lower your arm again, relaxing and opening your hand.

Repetitions: 5

This is a good exercise to use on an airplane when the decreased atmospheric pressure can causes swelling, especially since you can do it while seated.

Arm Stretches

Arm Raises

Doing arm raises will keep your shoulders flexible and will loosen that tight band sensation running down the inside of your arm. You can begin this stretch in the first week, but if the drain is still in, be sure you never lift your hands higher than your shoulders.

Position: Stand with your arms by your sides and your shoulders relaxed.

Motion: Keeping your arms straight, slowly raise both arms in front of you until your hands are level with your shoulders, palms facing the floor. Slowly, separate your arms until they're outstretched at your sides. Then, turn your palms up to face the ceiling. Finally, lower your arms to your sides.

Repetitions: 5

Back Climbing

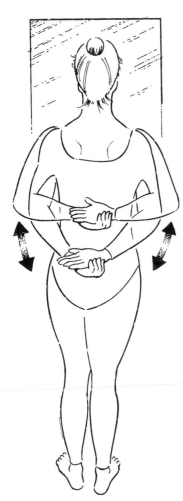

You may begin this exercise two weeks after your lumpectomy, after your drain is removed. You'll increase the flexibility in the muscles of your affected arm as you reach for the middle of your back.

Position: Stand straight.

Motion: Place your hands behind your lower back and clasp them together. Slowly slide your clasped hands up the center of your back. Stop when you start to feel your incision pulling. Hold that position for 15 seconds.

Repetitions: 1

Clasp-Lift Stretch

This stretch helps to increase the range of motion of your affected arm. Since you'll have to move your arms above shoulder level, don't attempt this until your drains are removed. Even if you did not have a drain, you should wait until the second week after surgery before you try this stretch.

Position: Stand upright.

Motion: Clasp your hands together in front of you. Slowly raise your hands toward the ceiling. Make sure your elbows are not bent, and your arms are straight. Stop when you feel your incision pulling. Hold that position for 15 seconds.

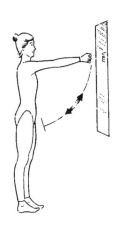

With your fingers still clasped, bend your arms and rest your clasped hands behind your head. Keep your head upright. Gradually extend your elbows back. Hold for 15 seconds.

Do this stretch daily. Each day that you repeat this exercise, you will find that you can move your clasped hands farther toward the back of your head. The first time you do the clasp-lift stretch, you may be able to touch only the upper part of your forehead. With each repetition, continue to challenge yourself by sliding your clasped hands a little farther over your head. Over time, you will eventually be able to move your clasped hands all the way to the back of your neck.

Repetitions: 1

Underarm Stretch

The purpose of this exercise is to stretch your underarm and the muscles in the back of your affected arm. As with the clasp-lift stretch, the underarm stretch should be done only after your drains are out or (if you have no drains) after the second week.

Position: Stand facing a wall.

Motion: Lift your affected arm as far as possible and lay your palm flat against the wall. Lean forward until you feel a stretch in your underarm area. Hold that position for 15 seconds. Return to an upright position and lower your arm. Do this stretch only once daily. Over time, you'll note improvement in your ability to stretch, and you can stand farther from the wall to start.

Repetitions: 1

Check Arm Flexibility

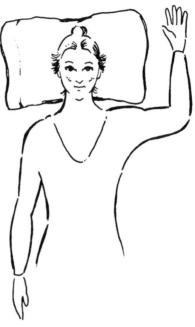

If you are scheduled for radiation therapy, you will be asked to lie on a treatment table with your arm extended to your side as shown in the illustration. At the end of the second week after your surgery, check your arm flexibility by lying on your bed with your arm extended in this position; it is the position that will be required for radiation therapy. If your arm is not flexible enough when the time for treatment arrives, the treatment may be delayed.

The exercises in this chapter should help you with range of motion so that you will be able to hold your arm in position without discomfort. However, if you think you need help, your surgeon can refer you to a physical therapist.

Upper Torso Stretches

Corner Stretches

To help stretch your chest muscles, you'll want to do corner stretches daily, beginning in the third week. This exercise should never be done when drains are in place.

Position: Stand facing the corner of the room.

Motion: With bent elbows, place the palms of your hands, thumbs down, against each side of the corner, so your forearms touch the walls and your elbows are at shoulder level.

Slowly lean forward, moving your chest toward the corner. Keep your elbows at shoulder level and your forearms flat against the wall as you lean in. You will feel the stretch across your chest. Hold this position for 15 seconds. Do this stretch only once daily.

Repetitions: 1

Weightlifting Exercises

Beginning in the third week and continuing throughout your recovery, some gentle weightlifting exercises will help build your arm muscles, keep them strong, and reduce your risk for lymphedema, a potentially chronic swelling caused by a collection of excess lymph fluid.

When all drains are removed and you are stretching on a daily basis, you should be ready for the slightly more strenuous weightlifting exercises, described in the pages ahead. To do them, you will need small weights, from one pound to five pounds. You may purchase them in any fitness or sports store and many department stores.

If you don't want to buy weights, you can start using some one-pound canned goods or small water bottles. Later, as you increase weight, partially-filled plastic water jugs can be substituted for weights.

Weightlifting exercises take about ten minutes and should be repeated every other day. You can combine or alternate them with stretching exercises. To avoid injury or overstraining, be sure to follow these guidelines:

- Use weights weighing five pounds or less. If you have previously used heavier weights and think you may be able to resume your previous routine, ask your hospital physical therapist for instruction.
- Perform these exercises only once a day, and never do them two days in a row. You'll be putting your muscles under some stress, and they need time to repair themselves.
- Stand erect in front of a mirror to check your form.
- Breathe correctly. Exhale with the effort, when you are lifting the weight. Inhale when you lower the weight and relax the muscle.

Shoulder Flexion

This weightlifting exercise works the deltoid muscle, which covers the upper part of your shoulder. This is the muscle flexed when you lift your arm overhead.

Position: Stand with your arms by your sides, holding weights comfortably in your hands. Your hands should be in a natural position, with the weights parallel to the floor.

Motion: Raise both arms evenly in front of your body, until both hands are directly overhead. As you perform this motion, keep your arms straight, and exhale.

Now lower your arms, reversing the same motion. Keep your arms straight as you bring them down directly in front of your body. Inhale as you slowly lower both arms.

Repetitions: 10

Biceps Curl

The biceps are upper arm muscles that help you lift your lower arm and hand. The biceps curl will help to return normal strength to that muscle.

Position: Stand with your arms by your sides, holding a weight in each hand.

Motion: Bending your arms, bring your hands (with the weights) as close to your shoulders as possible. Exhale as you perform this motion.

Slowly return your hands and arms to the starting position. Inhale.

Repetitions: 10

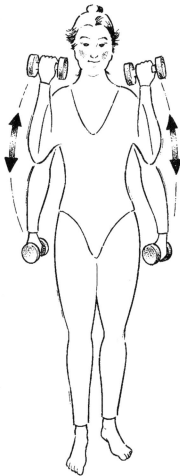

Arm Extension

This exercise strengthens the triceps muscle, which is under your upper arm, directly opposite the biceps. It's the muscle that helps you straighten the arm.

Position: Lie on your back on a mat or carpet, with your arms by your sides. Begin with a weight in your affected hand. Lift your lower arm from the floor by

bending your elbow and raising the weight until your lower arm is perpendicular to the floor. Hold the upper part of your weight-bearing arm with your opposite hand to steady your arm during the entire exercise.

Motion: Lift your whole arm from the floor, keeping the elbow bent, bringing the weight toward your shoulder until your elbow points toward the ceiling. Slowly straighten the arm until it is fully extended and your hand points toward the ceiling. Hold it for a few seconds. Exhale as you perform this motion. Slowly bring the weight toward your shoulder until your elbow points towards the ceiling. Inhale as you do so.

Repetitions: 10 on each side

Resuming Your Normal Activities

In six weeks your chest muscle will have healed completely. With daily stretching and strength training three times a week, you should regain your full arm mobility and strength. Normally, that's when you can resume sports that you enjoyed before surgery, such as golf, tennis, swimming, or running. Of course, your surgeon must give the okay before you resume aerobic exercise or return to a customary workout routine.

If you start chemotherapy, which usually begins three to four weeks after surgery, you'll probably experience the common, temporary side effect of fatigue. You may find that you don't have the stamina for strenuous exercise. Check with your doctors and nurses about continuing with a strenuous exercise program.

7

Radiation Therapy

Radiation therapy has been used to treat cancer for decades, and advances in modern medicine have made the treatment even more effective. The use of *computer tomography (CT)* in treatment planning, more sophisticated radiation therapy equipment, and treatment planning computers and software have made it possible to target the treatment area more precisely. As a result, other parts of the body, including the heart and lungs, are spared from significant amounts of radiation. The newer equipment is also more skin sparing; the skin is not permanently damaged as it was during treatment in the past.

As outlined previously, radiation therapy is routinely given after a lumpectomy for invasive breast cancer to reduce the risk of the cancer recurring in the breast. Like chemotherapy, radiation is effective in treating cancer because it kills fast-growing cells.

Meeting with Your Radiation Oncologist

In preparation for treatment, you will meet with a radiation oncologist, a physician who is specially trained to treat cancer with radiation therapy. During your first appointment, the radiation oncologist will perform a physical examination and review your medical history. He or she will explain the treatment process and discuss the risks and benefits. This is a good time to bring up any of your concerns. You may wish to ask such questions as:

- Why do you recommend radiation therapy for me?
- What are the common short-term side effects?
- What are the common long-term side effects?
- Will my heart or lungs be affected?
- What can be done to reduce the side effects?
- How long will each daily treatment last?
- How many weeks will the treatment take?

The Simulation Appointment

Before any treatments are given, you will be scheduled for a *simulation* or treatment planning appointment. The purpose of the simulation is to determine the precise *treatment field*—the parts of your breast and chest where the radiation beam will be aimed.

Once the treatment field is determined, the doctor or radiation therapist will mark your skin, creating a map of the area where radiation will be directed. They often mark key areas by tattooing tiny permanent blue dots, about the size of a pinhead, on your chest. They then will outline the treatment area with semi-permanent ink. Avoid washing off the ink while bathing until you are given the okay. (A word of caution: the ink can rub off on your clothes.)

During the simulation, the radiation specialists will also produce a customized mold, also referred to as an "immobility device," to hold your back and arm still and in exactly the same position in each treatment. Your simulation appointment will take one to two hours.

Radiation Treatments

Most courses of radiation treatment last six to eight weeks, with five treatments per week. Radiation therapy is delivered by a technician or therapist who operates a machine called a *linear accelerator*. Because the treatment is delivered externally, the form of treatment is known as *external beam radiation*.

When you receive a treatment, you will be asked to undress from the waist up and change into a hospital gown. Your therapist will ask you to lie on the treatment table with your customized mold under your back and arm. After you are carefully positioned under the machine, the therapist will leave the room and activate the equipment to deliver the radiation beam. (The therapist leaves the room each time to avoid exposure to radiation.) The actual treatment may take about a minute or two and is painless, much like an X-ray.

You will need to remain very still during the treatment. You don't have to hold your breath, nor should you breathe deeply—just breathe normally. Some women like to close their eyes and visualize that the radiation is sending a healing energy into their body.

Most women go through their radiation therapy with minimal side effects.

—Mark R.
radiation oncologist

You'll receive radiation therapy from two or more different angles. The therapist will reposition the machine for each treatment. When your daily treatment is over, your therapist will come back into the room. You'll be able to get dressed, leave, and carry on with your activities of the day.

Once a week, you'll meet with your radiation oncologist, who will check your progress. This is another opportunity to ask questions.

Radiation Boost Treatments

After you complete your five-week course of whole breast treatment, additional radiation may be administered to a smaller area where the tumor was located. This is called a *radiation boost* and is intended to eliminate any cancer cells that might remain around the area of the lumpectomy. The decision to use boost treatments is generally based on the size of the margin, the grade and size of the tumor, and age of the patient.

The radiation boost is commonly administered by external beam radiation. However, in some treatment centers, it is dispensed through internal radiation. The type of boost given depends mainly on the equipment the hospital has.

External Beam Boost Treatments

When you receive your external radiation boost treatment, you probably won't notice any difference in your treatment routine. You'll be treated in the same department and in a similar way as when you received your regular treatments. The only difference is that the radiation therapist will adjust the

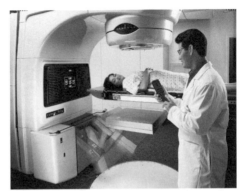

External beam radiation is delivered by a linear accelerator as shown above. Photo courtesy of Varian Medical Systems.

radiation equipment so that the field of radiation is smaller. The radiation boost treatments are generally administered daily for one to two weeks.

Internal Boost Treatments

Internal radiation, also called "brachytherapy," is a simple and safe procedure by which a radioactive implant is placed within the breast near the area where the tumor was located. The first part of the procedure requires the insertion of several very small tubes into your breast. This is performed in an operating room by your radiation oncologist, either at the time of your lumpectomy or in a separate procedure at the end of external radiation therapy. Since this is a fairly simple procedure, a local anesthesia is often sufficient; sometimes a general anesthesia is used.

The boost treatment begins when the radiation oncologist inserts tiny radioactive pellets into the tubes. These pellets transmit radiation into the area around your breast. There is usually no pain with this procedure, but sometimes, women feel slight discomfort.

The internal boost radiation may be given in low or high dose rates. Although the terms "low dose rate" and "high dose rate" suggest different levels of treatment, the two treatments are essentially the same. The difference is that the low dose rate brachytherapy is given on an inpatient basis and the high dose rate brachytherapy on an outpatient basis.

Low Dose Rate Boost Treatments

If you receive low dose rate boost treatments, the radiation implants remain in place for a day or two and you stay in the hospital.

After radiation treatment is finished, many women ask why they didn't experience fatigue. Most have only mild fatigue. Very few have extreme fatigue.

—Mark R.
Radiation oncologist

You will be asked to remain in your hospital room until the radioactive material is removed. Since the hospital staff works around radiation every day, an effort is made to reduce the amount of accumulated radiation they receive. So while your radioactive implant is in place, the hospital will limit the exposure of nurses and others who care for you. They will provide all your required care, but they will work quickly and speak to you from the doorway or over an intercom.

The hospital will also limit visitation. Children under age eighteen and pregnant women will not be allowed to visit. Visitors will be asked to sit at least six feet away and to limit their stay to less than one hour per day.

You should not feel pain or discomfort and will be able to move around the room freely. You'll be able to take care of your grooming needs, although you will be asked not to take a shower or get your implant wet.

Some patients report feeling a bit bored and lonely during this treatment period. Since you will be in the hospital for one to three days without much company, you may want to take along reading material or projects to pass the time.

After the completion of your internal radiation boost treatment, your radiation oncologist will remove the radioactive material and the tubes from your breast. Usually removal of the tubes is painless, and no anesthesia is required. After the radioactive material has been removed, it's perfectly safe for you to leave the hospital.

High Dose Rate Boost Treatments

If you having high dose rate boost radiation, you will be treated as an outpatient in the radiation therapy department. You will receive a daily treatment, which lasts a few minutes, over a period of several days. You will be taken to a treatment room where the radiation oncologist will insert small radioactive pellets into your thin breast tubes. In only a few minutes, your doctor will remove the radioactive implants.

At the end of the treatment session, you will be able to go home. After you receive the full course of treatments, the small tubes will be removed from your breast.

Side Effects of Radiation

Fatigue

During radiation treatments, your body will be working hard to kill cancer cells and to heal from the effects of treatment. One of the most common side effects is fatigue. Make an effort to stay well hydrated, as this flushes out the dead cells that radiation therapy kills and helps reduce fatigue. Plan to get extra rest. Take a short nap during the day, if you can, and get extra sleep at night.

Also continue to take daily walks, even if you are tired. As mentioned earlier, a half-hour walk every day during treatment will give you more energy. Also, keep up your exercises, particularly your stretching. If you stop stretching during radiation therapy, you will lose arm flexibility. A number of weeks after treatment ends, you'll probably notice that your energy level has returned to normal.

Skin Changes

Another predictable side effect of radiation is a temporary change in skin color and texture. Around the third week of treatment, your skin may show signs of redness and inflammation similar to sunburn. It may also become dry and feel warm, and an itchy rash may develop, but don't scratch it. Women with larger breasts typically suffer more of a skin reaction, and some women develop blisters in the fold on the underside of their breast and in the armpit area.

To minimize skin discomfort and speed healing, your nurse or doctor will give you instructions about special skin lotions to use. Use no other lotions on the treatment area. Other lotions may interfere with the delivery of the radiation.

Gently apply a thin coat of lotion to the whole treatment area, from underarm area to breastbone and from lower bra line up to collarbone. Also, include your shoulder, upper back, and neck. Apply the lotion after each daily treatment, after your bath or shower, and at bedtime, if you desire. Make sure that you do not apply the lotion within two hours before receiving your treatment. For example, if your treatment is at 10:00 A.M., do not apply your lotion after 8:00 A.M.

During radiation therapy, be gentle with the skin over the treated area. Here are some additional suggestions:

- Go without a bra.
- Wear soft, loose, clothing. Never wear tight clothing over the treated area.
- If your skin itches, apply a cool damp wash cloth.
- Do not rub, scrub, or scratch the skin.
- When you bathe or shower, use cool water to wash the treated area. Avoid using soap, which can irritate the skin. If you must, use a super fatty soap, such as Basis or unscented Dove.
- Avoid putting anything that is very hot on the area, such as a heating pad. You should never get in a hot tub or take a sauna while you're undergoing treatments.

- Do not apply anything cold, such as an ice pack, to the skin.
- Don't apply powders, creams, perfumes, or body oils that have not been recommended or approved by your nurse or doctor.
- Don't shave your underarm. If you must, use an electric razor.
- Avoid using deodorants or antiperspirants.
- Stay well hydrated.
- Avoid exposing the treated skin to sunshine. Wear protective clothing over the treated area when in daylight.

Other Short-Term Side Effects

Some women get a sore throat or dry cough when the treatment area is near the neck. If you do, tell your doctor about it. These symptoms usually go away a few weeks after treatment.

Weeks after treatment is over, some women develop a tiny fracture or irritation in a rib on the side that was treated. The fracture can cause discomfort, but it is not dangerous and does not require treatment. It heals on its own in a few weeks or months.

You may find that your breast feels sore and uncomfortable, particularly when your breast is examined or when you have a mammogram. Occasional soreness and moments of needle-like sensations may occur for months, or even years, after treatment. Slowly over time, the discomfort will diminish.

Possible Long-Term Side Effects

A few women experience some permanent long-term side effects. Your breast may look different. The pores on the breast skin might be larger, your breast may be slightly smaller, or larger, or your breast may appear more uplifted. The skin of the nipple and areola may feel slightly firmer. When you perform your self-examination, you may notice that your breast tissue feels smoother and slightly firmer.

Radiation injury to the heart or lungs is very uncommon. However, women who have radiation for left-sided breast cancer have a slightly higher risk of heart damage. Women who are treated with radiation therapy to the neck have a slightly higher risk of lung damage. Radiation therapy to the underarm or the neck has a slightly higher risk of causing lymphedema.

What Is Partial Breast Irradiation?

Partial breast irradiation (PBI) is a topic you may be hearing more about. It is currently under investigation as a new treatment method that treats only part of the breast with radiation, rather than the whole breast. This treatment minimizes radiation exposure to healthy tissue, and the treatment takes only about five days, rather than several weeks. It can also be delivered prior to chemotherapy, which may provide additional protection against recurrence.

> *Three things helped me the most: I had a friend go with me to daily treatments. I applied cream to my skin three times a day, and I used visualization.*
>
> — Nora, 57

Who is a candidate for PBI? Generally, good candidates are thought to be women with smaller tumors who have clear surgical margins, have only one site of disease, and have no lymph node involvement. Several different techniques are being evaluated around the world including both internal and external delivery of radiation.

How effective is the treatment? Early results are promising. A five-year study compared several hundred women, half of whom had full-breast radiation therapy; the other half had PBI. The group that had PBI had no higher rate of recurrence, and survival rates for both groups were the same. In the fall of 2003, the National Cancer Institute began a large-scale study to further study the long-term effectiveness of partial breast irradiation.

8

Chemotherapy and Hormonal Therapy

Over the years, you've probably known women who have gone through chemotherapy or hormonal therapy. If they were relatives or close friends, you probably helped them during their treatment. Even so, you were on the outside, observing someone else's cancer treatment. But now, perhaps you're the one considering the treatment—chemotherapy or hormonal therapy may be recommended after your lumpectomy.

Most women initially faced the prospect of chemotherapy with fear and dread. But times have changed. Today, most women who have gone through chemotherapy will tell you that it was not as bad as they expected. Newer medications are effective in minimizing side effects, and many women continue to work during their treatment.

How Chemotherapy Works

Chemotherapy is often referred to as *adjuvant therapy*, which simply means additional or supporting therapy. It is a *systemic therapy*—the chemotherapy agents circulate throughout the entire system. How does chemotherapy work? Chemotherapy kills rapidly reproducing cells, because cells are most vulnerable when they are reproducing. Cancer cells multiply rapidly, so the chemotherapy agents destroy them. Fast-growing normal cells are also harmed and this causes many of the side effects of chemotherapy. Since normal cells are capable of repairing themselves, the side effects are temporary.

When Is Chemotherapy Needed?

After your lumpectomy, your doctors will be in a better position to judge how your treatment plan should be individualized. Several factors are taken into consideration, including your surgeon's observation during surgery, a careful analysis of the tissue removed during surgery (the pathology report), your general health, and possibly results from other tests such as chest X-ray, bone scan, and MRI and CT scans.

Consultation with the Medical Oncologist

Having chemotherapy is an important decision, so it's essential to have a medical oncologist who is highly qualified. You want a doctor who will spend time with you, make sure your questions are answered, and put you at ease. Your surgeon will probably recommend a medical oncologist. Make sure the oncologist has the following qualifications:

- Board certification in medical oncology. This means that the doctor has passed rigorous examinations.
- Extensive experience in treatment of breast cancer. You can get this information from your own surgeon, from other breast cancer survivors, or from local advocacy groups.

You may want to take a spouse or friend with you to this appointment to listen, take notes, and ask questions. It may be helpful to make a list of any questions you have and take it to your appointment. You may wish to ask such questions as:

- What is my prognosis without chemotherapy? What is my prognosis with chemotherapy?
- Do you recommend chemotherapy? What medications do you suggest?
- How many treatments will I need?
- How often will I come in for treatments?
- Where will I receive my treatments?

- How long will each treatment session last?
- What are the common side effects of chemotherapy?
- What can be done to reduce the side effects?
- Will I be able to work while on chemotherapy?

Seeking a Second Opinion

During your first visit to a medical oncologist, you need not make a decision about your treatment. Many women need time to think about what was said during the appointment. It might be helpful to get a second opinion. Your medical oncologist will not feel offended if you seek a second opinion. To the contrary, doctors want you to feel that you are making the best personal choice.

Under what circumstances might a second opinion be helpful? In general, it's always a good idea to talk to more than one medical oncologist. Opinions on the types and combinations of medications, the length and frequency of treatment, and the benefit of chemotherapy and hormonal therapy vary among medical oncologists. And as previously mentioned, you may also want to get a second pathology review, since an accurate and complete pathology report is essential. Some larger centers offer a formal second opinion service, in which your pathology slides are sent to expert pathologists for interpretation and you have a consultation with a medical oncologist.

Many times, a second opinion confirms the findings of the first doctor. If you find, however, that the second opinion is substantially different, you may actually need a third opinion.

If you see another doctor, you will need to take copies of your pathology report as well as any other test results from blood work and

> *During chemo take your anti nausea medication regularly. This always keeps the medication in your blood stream. You feel so much better when you do this.*
>
> *— Edith, 64*

X-rays. It is wise to have personal copies of all these reports; you may ask the medical oncologist or your surgeon for copies.

How Chemotherapy Is Administered

If you are to receive chemotherapy, you will receive your treatments in your doctor's office or in your hospital's infusion center. The session will likely last one to three hours. You'll probably be seated in a comfortable reclining chair. Ask for a pillow or light blanket if you need it. For your first treatment, you might feel better if a friend or relative goes along; you may have less anxiety if a loved one stays with you.

Chemotherapy is given on a set schedule. Most commonly, it's administered every twenty-one days, although sometimes it is given every two weeks or even weekly. Treatments usually continue from four to eight months.

Chemotherapy is usually delivered intravenously by IV. Medical personnel call this a "drip," since the medication drips from a hanging bottle into your IV. Your oncology nurse or doctor will start an IV in your hand or arm opposite the side of your surgery. You will first receive some hydrating fluids, then powerful anti-nausea medication. When you are well medicated, which may make you feel sleepy, you will be given chemotherapy. It's important to hold your hand and arm still so that the IV stays in your vein.

When your treatment is over, your nurse will remove your IV. You should feel fine. However, it is best to go home right after your treatment so that you can rest.

Before you leave, make sure you have the name and phone number of someone to call with questions. If you have any concerns about managing your care at home, don't hesitate to call. Make sure that your nurse has given you a written list of your anti-nausea medications and an explanation of how and when to take them.

Chemotherapy Agents

Six chemotherapy agents are commonly given as adjuvant therapy for breast cancer:

- cyclophosphamide (Cytoxan)
- methotrexate (M)
- 5-fluorouracil (F)
- adriamycin (A)
- epirubicin (E)
- paclitaxel (Taxol) (T)
- docetaxel (Taxotere) (T)

These chemotherapy drugs are usually given in combinations, such as CMF, AC, ACT, FEC, or AC followed by T.

Side Effects of Chemotherapy

Chemotherapy is likely to produce a number of well-known side effects, such as nausea, hair loss, and fatigue. Some women say they feel like they have a bad flu for about three to five days after each treatment; however, many women find that side effects are not as bad as they feared. Many women feel well enough to work during their course of chemotherapy.

Nausea and Vomiting

The nausea associated with chemotherapy has a predictable rhythm. Since you'll be given anti-nausea medications at the time of your treatment, you'll probably feel okay for the first twenty-four hours. The next morning, however, you're likely to begin experiencing nausea and possibly vomiting. Many women say these side effects peak on the third day. After that, you'll probably start feeling better.

For many women, nausea is the most dreaded result of chemotherapy treatments. However, improved ways of administering chemotherapy and new anti-nausea medications make severe nausea and vomiting the exception, not the rule.

Drop in Blood Count

Your *bone marrow* produces your platelets, white blood cells (WBC), and red blood cells (RBC). These rapidly growing cells are harmed by chemotherapy so that your *blood count* is temporarily lowered. *Platelets* help blood clot. When your platelets are low, you will bruise more easily and you might notice bleeding gums if you brush your teeth vigorously. *White blood cells* fight infection, and *red blood cells* carry oxygen to cells.

In most patients, the blood count plummets to its lowest level some seven to ten days after each treatment. This lowest point is called the *nadir.* Since your WBCs play an important role in fighting infections, when you are at your nadir, your immune system will be weakened and you will be susceptible to viruses and bacteria.

Fatigue

Most people begin to feel tired after their first chemotherapy treatment. This fatigue generally continues throughout your treatment. One reason for this is the chemotherapy's effects on red blood cells. Consequently, when your red blood cells are at their nadir, they are not delivering oxygen efficiently, and you will feel very tired. This condition is called chemotherapy-induced anemia. It will temporarily, but dramatically, add to your fatigue. When you are at your nadir, you may also notice that you have shortness of breath when you exercise or walk up stairs.

If your RBCs stay low and you are very tired, your doctor may recommend a medication, like *Procrit,* which stimulates the production of RBCs. Some women have remarkable results from such medications, so be sure to ask your doctor about them.

As previously discussed, walking daily can help maintain your energy, so continue walking even if you are tired. At the same time, it's important to conserve energy. Decide what is really important for you to do and what you should let go of. If you work at a full-time job, perhaps you can reduce the number of hours you work during a course of therapy.

Hair Loss

The most obvious physical side effect of chemotherapy is temporary hair thinning or hair loss. Since all hair is made up of fast-growing cells, the hair on your scalp, as well as your eyebrows, eyelashes, and pubic hair will be affected by the chemotherapy agents.

Most women begin to lose hair from their scalp around the nineteenth day after the first chemotherapy treatment. Your scalp will start feeling tender a few days before your hair falls out, and once it does, it usually comes out rapidly—within the following two to three days. For many women, this is an emotionally devastating experience. Many women say that losing their hair was as traumatic to them as being diagnosed with breast cancer. But remember that after treatment, all of your hair will grow back.

To help cope with hair loss, you have many resources, including eye make-up, hairpieces, hats, and scarves. To shape your eyebrows, try an eyebrow powder, which creates a more natural brow line than an eyebrow pencil.

The key to a natural looking and attractive hairpiece is to have it professionally cut and styled while it's on your head. Consider buying a synthetic wig. They are easy to take care of (they require only shampooing), and many are priced under $300.00. A wig made of human hair may seem desirable, but it's often impractical. The human hair needs constant shampooing, blow-drying, and curling. The cost is nearly four times that of a synthetic wig. Unfortunately, most insurance companies do not cover the cost of hairpieces. If your insurance does, make sure that you get a doctor's prescription for a cranial prosthesis.

Menopausal Symptoms

Chemotherapy may create chemically induced menopause. This occurs in 10 to 50 percent of women younger than forty and in 50 to 94 percent of women over forty. It occurs because women's ovaries are made up of fast-growing cells, so chemotherapy agents affect them. A woman's period usually stops during treatment. If you're under forty, your period may return, but the closer you are to menopause, the less likely your periods will return.

Take chemo one day at a time. Don't be hard on yourself, and most of all, don't be afraid to ask for help.

—Linda, 58

Other menopausal symptoms include hot flashes, night sweats, and vaginal dryness. The frequency and intensity of hot flashes generally lessen over time, although that may take many months. If you're having hot flashes, you may wish to review the coping suggestions listed later on in this chapter. If you are troubled by vaginal dryness your doctor can prescribe estrogen by vaginal suppository. Don't worry; only a very small amount gets absorbed systemically, so it is perfectly safe to use even if your tumor is estrogen positive.

Many women report a lessening of sexual desire during treatment. This is generally temporary. After the completion of chemotherapy, give yourself several months to regain interest in sex. If there's no change, you may wish to speak with your doctor; one possibility is that your testosterone levels are diminished, a side effect of chemotherapy. Many counselors are specially trained to talk with you about sexual intimacy and can suggest steps to enhance sexual desire.

Memory Loss

Many women notice that while on chemotherapy, they develop problems with short-term memory and concentration. This is often referred to as "chemo brain." But reactions vary. Some women experience no memory problems; others encounter so much memory loss that it actually interferes with daily life. In addition to the chemotherapy itself, memory problems might be aggravated by stress, fatigue, anti-anxiety medications, and the onset of menopause. Any or all of these factors can negatively affect memory. Be patient with yourself and compensate for it; for example, focus on one task or one conversation at a time, and make and use lists. When chemotherapy is over, most women who have experienced "chemo brain" find that their memory improves.

Weight Loss

Some women lose weight during chemotherapy. This may occur for several reasons. Immediately after treatments, some women say they have a metallic taste in their mouths, some women have an extra sensitivity to smells and tastes, and some women are bothered by mouth sores. All this does improve in time. Meanwhile, however, it can be challenging to find something to eat or drink that tastes and feels good. Your emotional state also affects your appetite; anxiety and depression can cause anorexia.

Some women are pleased to be losing weight, but it is important to take in enough calories to help your body rebuild the tissue damaged during treatment. If you continue to lose weight, ask your medical oncologist to refer you to a hospital dietician. If anxiety and depression are reducing your appetite, ask for a referral to a mental health professional.

Weight Gain

Far more women find that they gain weight during treatment, particularly during chemotherapy. This occurs for several reasons. Feeling fatigued, many women cut back on their exercise and physical activity. Chemotherapy can cause menopause and menopause itself can cause weight gain. Some women find that eating regularly, particularly carbohydrates, soothes the stomach and reduces nausea. Other women find comfort in food. Food can be an important source of pleasure during this difficult time. So if you find that you are gaining weight, be patient. It may be more realistic to wait until treatment is over to begin a healthy weight loss program.

Other Possible Side Effects

Some chemotherapy patients report digestive side effects such as heartburn, gas, diarrhea, and constipation. Your entire digestive system is lined in fast-growing cells that are affected by chemotherapy. If you have any of these side effects, do not self-medicate or suffer in silence. Call your doctor or nurse.

Some women develop mouth sores that look and feel like cold sores. They occur because the mucous lining of the mouth is made up of fast-growing cells. You can reduce your risk of mouth sores by avoiding commercial mouthwashes—they are too harsh and drying. Instead, use a gentler mouthwash by combining one quart of water, one teaspoon of salt, and one teaspoon of baking soda. Use this before going to bed at night and after each meal. If you do develop mouth sores, your doctor can prescribe a numbing mouthwash or a salve that helps reduce the discomfort.

Tips for Managing Side Effects

Drink Fluids

Be sure to drink plenty of hydrating liquids (eight to ten glasses), particularly the day before, the day of, and the three days after chemotherapy. In addition to reducing nausea, fluids flush out the byproducts of chemotherapy and protect your bladder from the chemotherapy toxins. Chemotherapy can affect your sense of taste, so if plain water is not to your liking, experiment with different flavors, consistencies, and temperatures. Try diluted fruit juice, ginger ale or ginger root tea, or Gatorade. Try something cold like popsicles, ice chips or sorbets. Warm beverages such as low-salt broths or herbal teas may be soothing. Fruits, particularly watermelon, are hydrating, too.

Take Anti-Nausea Medications

Take your anti-nausea medications on a fixed schedule. Using your medications effectively is key to keeping your nausea under control. Most women need a combination of anti-nausea medications. Medications typically come in three forms: a pill that's taken orally with water, a dissolving pill to be placed under your tongue, or a rectal suppository. Ask your nurse to help you understand exactly how to use the different medications and write down the schedule for you. The most commonly used anti-nausea medications are:

- Zofran, Kytril or Anzement
- Compazine
- Ativan
- Decadron

If you are vomiting repeatedly, call your doctor. Your doctor may prescribe a different oral medication. Or your doctor may suggest a rectal suppository—most commonly Compazine—which usually works well to stop vomiting. Your doctor may also prescribe Ativan, an anti-nausea and anti-anxiety medication, that is placed under your tongue.

Vomiting causes dehydration, so take in liquids as soon as possible. If you have gone thirty minutes without vomiting, start hydrating with ice chips. After tolerating ice chips for half an hour, take a tablespoon of water every ten minutes. Thirty minutes later, you should be able to start sipping water. Staying well hydrated helps reduce the cycle of nausea and vomiting.

If these suggestions do not work, then it is important to call your doctor or oncology nurse again. Sometimes you may need IV hydration and IV anti-nausea medication, which requires a visit to your doctor's office, the emergency room, or an infusion center. Severe dehydration can be a life-threatening emergency, and it is important to get appropriate medical care as soon as possible.

Eat Small Meals

Eat for comfort. Small, frequent meals every two and a half to three hours are usually preferable to three large meals or nothing at all. When eating seems difficult, choose what appeals to you, even if it is not the most healthy. Carbohydrates seem to work the best, such as potatoes, macaroni and cheese, rice pudding, ice cream, rice, bagels, and toast. Though you may not have much appetite, many women find that eating just a little bit helps calm the stomach.

Avoid foods that typically irritate the stomach such as spicy or fried foods, citrus fruits (oranges and grapefruit), caffeine, alcohol, and peppermint.

Try to Relax

Feeling relaxed and comfortable also helps you manage nausea. When you're resting, you want a quiet, cool room with dim lighting. Open a window to let in some fresh air. It helps to lie down with a pillow under your head and torso so that they are slightly elevated.

Get Plenty of Rest

Try to get a good night's sleep every night. This may be a challenge, because chemotherapy itself and medications such as *Decadron* (for nausea), may make it difficult for you to fall asleep and to stay asleep. Ativan not only reduces nausea and anxiety, it helps you fall asleep and stay asleep at night. So don't hesitate to use this or any other sleep medication your doctor prescribes.

Monitor Your Blood Count

During chemotherapy, your medical oncologist will carefully monitor your blood count by taking a small sample of your blood with a finger prick. Your body has an amazing capacity to heal, and your blood count will start rising again after each chemotherapy treatment.

If your WBCs remain at a low level, you may need a medication that stimulates bone marrow, such as Neupogen. Your medical oncologist will be able to tell you whether you can benefit from such a medication.

I found it comforting that my husband was able to accompany me to the chemo treatments, even if we both dozed off once in a while.

Sarah, 57

Guard Against Infections

Since the cold virus is very common, you'll be susceptible to upper respiratory infections, particularly during your nadir. During the few days of your nadir, avoid crowds, public transportation, airplane travel, going to the gym, and the company of young children, as children tend to get a lot of colds.

If you have cold symptoms—sneezing, congestion, or runny nose—start taking your temperature three times a day. If you do get a fever, or feel very ill, call your medical oncologist's office immediately. If your doctor is not available, go to the nearest hospital emergency

---

Washing Hands to Kill Germs

- Wet hands and apply soap.

- Wash the backs of hands as well as palms.

- Rub vigorously to remove bacteria that stick to skin.

- Wash vigorously for twenty seconds.

---

room. When your WBC count is very low, you can become very ill very fast.

During your nadir you are at increased risk of bladder infections and vaginal yeast infections. A bladder infection is signaled by an urgent need to urinate frequently and a burning sensation when you do. You can help avoid getting a bladder infection by staying well hydrated to keep the bladder flushed, and by wiping from front to back after each bowel movement to avoid contaminating the urethra. A yeast infection is indicated by burning or itching and a vaginal discharge. If you get the symptoms of either bladder or yeast infection, call your doctor immediately or go to an emergency room so that you can be started on an appropriate treatment.

Studies have shown that the most effective way to reduce your risk of catching a cold is simply by washing your hands frequently and thoroughly with hot water and soap. Wash your hands as often as possible, especially after going to the bathroom, before eating, and before going to bed at night.

Hormonal Therapy

Hormonal therapy, also called endocrine therapy, is used to prevent the growth or recurrence of breast cancer. To better understand how this therapy works, let's first examine how natural hormones stimulate the growth of some breast cancers.

When cancer cells are analyzed in a pathology lab, pathologists can determine whether the cancer is stimulated by the female hormones estrogen and progesterone. If so, the tumors are referred to as estrogen positive or progesterone positive.

Even after menopause, a woman's body still makes estrogen. So when tumors are estrogen positive, one of two types of hormone therapy may be recommended. One form, called a *selective estrogen receptor modulator (SERM)*, attaches to cancer cells and prevents them from growing. Tamoxifen works this way. The second, newer therapeutic agents, called *armatase inhibitors,* block the production of estrogen throughout the body thereby essentially starving the cancer cells.

Hormonal therapy may be given in place of chemotherapy or in addition to it. Hormonal therapy may replace chemotherapy when the lymph nodes are negative, the tumor is small and slow growing, and the tumor is estrogen positive. Hormonal therapy is routinely given in addition to chemotherapy when a woman has a tumor that is estrogen positive and she meets other criteria for chemotherapy; for example, the cancer has spread into lymph nodes.

Tamoxifen Therapy

The most commonly used hormonal therapy is *tamoxifen*. More than twenty years of data show that tamoxifen extends the lifespan of many breast cancer patients. An oral medication, tamoxifen, (*Nolvadex*) is taken in pill form for five years. The treatment decreases the risk of cancer recurrence in the breast and in other organs. Studies have also shown that women who have had cancer in one breast, have a significantly reduced risk of cancer in the other breast when taking tamoxifen.

Side Effects of Tamoxifen

Hormonal therapy is much gentler than chemotherapy, and produces significantly fewer and milder side effects. Still, tamoxifen may bring on menopausal symptoms such as hot flashes and night sweats. These generally improve over time. Some women report vaginal dryness or vaginal discharge. Other possible side effects include:

- weight gain
- slight increase in the risk of blood clots
- slight increase in the risk of uterine cancer
- increased depression for those with a history of depression

Other Hormonal Treatments

The newer hormonal treatments, known as *aromatase inhibitors,* act differently than Tamoxifen. They block a woman's body from making estrogen. The drugs (anastrozole) *Arimidex,* (letrozole) *Femara,* and (exemestane) *Aromasin* block estrogen production in postmenopausal women. Some women who take aromatase inhibitors have reported joint pain and stiffness. There is also an increased incidence of osteoporosis and of bone fractures. However, when compared to tamoxifen, aromatase inhibitors show a lower incidence of such side effects as endometrial cancer and blood clots.

The drugs, goserelin (*Zoladex*) and leuprolide acetate (*Lupron*) suppress ovarian estrogen production in premenopausal women. They cause menopausal symptoms such as hot flashes and vaginal dryness.

Managing Hot Flashes

If you are troubled by hot flashes during the day and at night, you can take a number of steps that may reduce their frequency or intensity. Here are a few suggestions:

- Avoid certain foods that are known to trigger hot flashes, such as caffeine, alcohol, and spicy foods.
- Avoid hot tubs, saunas, hot baths, hot showers, and hot beverages. In hot weather, try to stay cool.
- Dress in layers. If you wear a sleeveless shirt under a sweater or jacket, you can quickly remove the outer layer and immediately feel more comfortable. Avoid turtleneck shirts or sweaters.
- Stay well hydrated.

- Take a daily thirty-minute walk.
- Sleep in a cold room at night, under light covers, in a light, sleeveless nightgown and no socks.

Gynecological Care

It's important to see your gynecologist routinely, at least once a year. If you are taking hormonal therapy, your gynecologist needs to be particularly attentive to signs of uterine cancer. One warning sign is unexplained vaginal bleeding.

Anyone with a strong family history of breast cancer should be monitored for indications of ovarian cancer. A strong family history means that multiple relatives in multiple generations, from either side of your family, have had breast and/or ovarian cancer.

In addition to discussing your family history with your gynecologist, you may also want to meet with a medical geneticist, who is trained to help you and your doctors determine if you are, in fact, at higher risk for ovarian cancer. Although there are no obvious warnings signs of ovarian cancer, a vaginal ultrasound is helpful in screening for both uterine and ovarian cancer, and may be recommended by your gynecologist.

9

Nutrition: Healthful Eating

Good nutrition is essential for good health. It is especially important to eat health-promoting foods when your body is recovering from surgery or treatment for cancer. A nutrient-rich diet helps maintain your strength and prevents body tissue from breaking down. It also helps rebuild tissues that may have been harmed during chemotherapy or radiation treatments.

In addition to helping you recover from treatment, good nutrition *may* help combat cancer. Currently, there is not enough scientific evidence to prove that specific foods cause cancer or prevent it, but comprehensive studies by major health organizations have published nutritional guidelines, that, if followed, may lower one's risk of cancer.

An "Anti-Cancer" Diet

Nutritional guidelines from both the American Institute for Cancer Research and the American Cancer Society suggest that a cancer-fighting food plan should include a variety of plant-based foods—at least five servings of fruits and vegetables daily, along with beans, nuts, seeds, and whole grains. Fish and skinless poultry are recommended in place of red meat.

Why a diet rich in plant-based foods? These foods contain compounds called "phytonutrients", plant nutrients that seem to boost the body's natural defenses against *carcinogens*—that is, cancer-causing substances. Populations dependent on plant-based diets have a lower rate of certain cancers, suggesting that their intake of phytonutrients seems to combat carcinogens and help protect cells from damage.

You can increase the proportion of phytonutrients in your diet without making radical lifestyle changes. In fact, your best resource is no farther away than your nearest supermarket. There is, however, one particular food that is generally underutilized in the American diet, and it seems to provide special benefits as a cancer fighter.

That food is soy.

The Japanese Diet—A Special Case

For some time, medical researchers have been intrigued by studies showing that Japanese women, whose diets are high in soy, have a significantly lower risk of breast cancer than American women. Natural products made from soybeans include soymilk, tofu, tempeh, edamame (whole green soybean), and soy nut (baked soybean), all of which are prominent in the traditional Japanese diet. The incidence of breast cancer among Japanese women is 5 per 100,000. America's rate is 22.4 per 100,000. A Japanese woman has about one-fourth the risk of getting breast cancer as an American woman.

I can't stress enough how important it is to have good nutrition and get plenty of rest.

— Patricia Ann, 57

It is important to keep in mind that the traditional Japanese diet also includes many other plant-based foods, among them green tea, seaweed, and maitake and shiitake mushrooms (which most Americans don't eat). Their diet also includes a high proportion of fish, whereas Americans tend to eat more red meat. Japanese women consume little alcohol and almost no processed foods or hydrogenated oils, used in many processed foods like commercially baked goods. But even when these differences are taken into account, researchers think it's likely that soybeans have a special component that helps reduce breast cancer risk.

Recommended Sources of Carbohydrates

Current nutritional guidelines suggest that most Americans should be getting more vegetables, fruits, and whole grains in their diets. All these foods contain complex carbohydrates. When you eat them, you unlock rich sources of vitamins and minerals that help protect your body cells and improve the way your organs function.

Unprocessed fruits, vegetables, grains, beans, nuts and seeds offer other benefits. These foods are high in fiber. Studies have shown that groups of people on high-fiber diets tend to have a lower incidence of colon cancer, heart disease, and other health problems than people who consume diets lower in fiber.

Cruciferous Vegetables

Studies have consistently found that people who eat cruciferous vegetables, members of the cabbage family, have a lower risk of cancer, particularly breast cancer. The compound in these vegetables that seems to be the chief cancer fighter is indole-3 carbinol.

Indole-3 carbinol and other compounds stimulate detoxification in the body—that is, they remove and or deactivate harmful substances that can cause cell damage. Numerous animal and cell culture studies show that indole-3 is a potent antagonist of breast cancer cells.

Cruciferous Vegetables with Indole-3 Carbinol

- Bok choy
- Broccoli
- Brussels sprouts
- Cabbage
- Radish
- Kale
- Mustard seed
- Rutabaga
- Turnip
- Watercress

Carbohydrate Sources to Avoid

When you eat simple carbohydrates—white bread, pasta, white rice, packaged cereals, rice cakes, crackers, cookies, and cakes—you're missing the benefits you get from nutrient-rich foods. Packaged and processed foods contribute little to your health, and many are harmful to the extent that they cause weight gain and blood sugar problems.

How so? Once digested, these foods become sugar in the body and stimulate the production of insulin. In turn, the body coverts the sugar into fat and stores it, which adds to your supply of body fat. Our fat makes and stores estrogen, and studies show that being overweight may increase the risk of breast cancer. In addition, we do know that obesity increases our risk for many other diseases, particularly heart disease and diabetes.

So it's important to think about the carbohydrates you choose. When you have an apple, figs, or a handful of almonds for a snack instead of crackers, or cookies, or chips, you're giving your body a nutrient-rich reward of complex carbohydrates rather than empty calories that raise your blood sugar level and contribute to weight gain.

Recommended Sources of Protein

Protein is essential to repair tissue damage from surgery, chemotherapy, and radiation therapy, and it should be part of your diet every day. Protein can be found in both plant and animal food sources. Although many people think of red meat as a prime source of protein, there are other, more healthful sources as well; fish, beans, and raw nuts and seeds among them.

Many studies have shown that vegetarians have a lower rate of all kinds of cancers and most diseases (heart disease, diabetes, and osteoporosis) compared with people who eat a lot of red meat and poultry. Beans—such as, soybeans, black beans, garbanzo beans, red beans, and kidney beans—and raw nuts and seeds are delicious and healthy sources of plant protein. They are also high in fiber and contain no saturated fat, so they do not increase your risk of heart disease.

Protein from Fish

In countries where people eat a lot of deep-water and cold-water fish, the populations usually have a decreased incidence of both cancer and heart disease. Fish is an excellent source of protein. It also has a kind of fat called omega-3 that seems to be a cancer-fighting agent.

Fish is also rich in vitamin D, a nutrient found to help ward off breast cancer in postmenopausal women. If you enjoy eating fish, you may eat it daily. However, be aware that some fish have been found to contain mercury, which can cause neurological toxicity at high levels. Fortunately, some of the healthiest fish and seafood have the lowest mercury levels. Salmon, sardines, mackerel, herring, halibut, cod, anchovies, striped bass, trout, oyster, and squid contain low levels of mercury and high levels of omega-3. Avoid a daily tuna sandwich since tuna, mahi mahi, and swordfish contain high mercury levels and should be eaten no more than once a week.

Eat protein, drink a lots of water, moisturize your skin, and hug some you love.

—Karen, 46

Meats in Moderation

Most of us find that meats such as steak, hamburger, and chicken are hard to give up. The solution is to cut back on portion size. For a nutritional balance and plenty of protein, all you need are three ounces (after cooking) of red meat or poultry per serving. That serving is just about the size of the palm of your hand. If you're accustomed to more than that, the reduced portion may look small. But if you fill the rest of your plate with the recommended servings of plant foods, you'll be getting a satisfying and tasty meal that's much more healthful.

Protein from Dairy Products

Milk, yogurt, cheese, and other dairy products are another source of protein, but these foods are high in saturated fat. However, as long as you select nonfat daily products, you get the protein content without the saturated fat, which contributes to weight gain, diabetes, and heart disease.

Protein Sources to Avoid

Most lunchmeats, ham, and hot dogs are preserved with nitrites to maintain color and prevent contamination with bacteria. However, nitrites turn into carcinogenic nitrosamines in your stomach. If you enjoy sandwiches, replace processed lunchmeats with canned salmon or slices of fresh chicken, turkey, or roast beef. A diet high in fruits and vegetables contains vitamin C and other photochemicals, such as phenols, which retard the conversion of nitrites to nitrosamines.

Grilled meats may be particularly harmful to health. Studies show that if you barbecue, broil, or pan-fry meat at high heat, the cooking process introduces heterocyclic amines, which may contribute to cancer development. Animal studies have shown that heterocyclic amines damage the genetic material inside cells and induce tumors.

Meats that are boiled, stewed, or poached have fewer harmful substances, particularly if the meat is cooked rare to medium. If you like grilling and want to reduce the presence of the carcinogenic substances, you can microwave meat or poultry for two to five minutes before putting it on the grill. That releases juices that contain precursors of heterocyclic amines. (Be sure to discard the juice.) Or you can marinate the meat before grilling in a marinade that has lots of lemon or lime juice. The marinade reduces the presence of carcinogens.

Recommended Sources of Fat

Fat is often misunderstood. For years, doctors and nutritionists advocated a low-fat diet to help us lose weight and improve our blood cholesterol levels. This point is well taken, since most of us consume too much fat. However, we all need *some* fat as part of good nutrition. We can't live without it. Fats keep cell membranes fluid and flexible.

They promote growth of cells, blood vessels, and nerves, and they keep skin and other tissues lubricated.

However, not all fats are alike. The good fats are unsaturated fats, and there are two categories of these:

- Polyunsaturated fats, found in fish and plant sources
- Monounsaturated fats, found in oils such as olive and canola

Healthful Polyunsaturated Fats

Particularly desirable polyunsaturated fats are those found in the cold-water fish like salmon and sardines—omega-3 fats, an essential fatty acid. Studies have shown that the omega-3s improve the ratio of "good cholesterol" (HDL) high-density lipids to "bad cholesterol" (LDL) low-density lipids, so they benefit arterial health. And as previously stated, omega-3 fats have cancer-fighting properties as well.

Plant sources of omega-3 fats include flaxseed, soybeans, walnuts, oat germ, raw spinach, wheat germ, and raw broccoli. Flaxseed is a rich source of alpha-liolenic acids, one of the omega-3 fats. It also has a beneficial type of fiber called *lignans*. Studies have shown that both alpha-liolenic acid and lignans offer protection against breast cancer. So if you don't enjoy fish, supplement your diet with two tablespoons of ground flaxseed a day. The tiny flaxseeds must be ground to release the oil, but the oil is quite perishable and heat destroys it. Refrigerate it and sprinkle it raw on cold foods. Ground flaxseed has a pleasant nutty taste.

Fish High in Omega-3 Fats

- Mackerel, Atlantic
- Trout, lake
- Herring, Atlantic
- Salmon, Atlantic
- Halibut
- Cod

Healthful Monounsaturated Fats

Olive oil is an excellent monounsaturated fat because it is an *antioxidant*. Antioxidants protect against heart disease and reduce the risk of cancer. Studies show that populations consuming a lot of olive oil—Spain, Italy, and Greece—have a lower rate of breast cancer than American women. Greek women have one-third the incidence of breast cancer as American women. Learn to appreciate olive oil in your cooking and in your salads. Use virgin or extra virgin, cold-pressed olive oil; these varieties are made from the first pressing of the olive and are nutritionally richer.

Canola oil is another monounsaturated fat. Think of it as a neutral oil, it has a neutral taste, and although it does not contain beneficial antioxidants, it is not harmful for your heart or your general health.

Fats to Avoid

In the last thirty years consumers have increased their consumption of artificial fats. The increased consumption of bad fats has, without a doubt, contributed to the incidence of heart disease. Some research suggests that the wrong types of fats may contribute to the development of cancer. Bad fats include:

- *Saturated fats* are mainly found in animal fats, whole-milk products, and some plants. Foods, including coconut and coconut oil, palm oil, and palm kernel oil.
- *Trans fats* act like saturated fats. They are produced by heating vegetable oil to a solid state to extend the shelf life of food products, a process known as hydrogenation. The more solid the fat, the more trans fats. These hydrogenated fats are found in commercially prepared baked goods, margarine, snack foods, and processed foods. Commercially fried foods, such as French fries, are high in trans fats.

Another type of fat, the omega-6 fats, come from such foods as vegetable oils and the meat of grain-fed animals. Too much of these fats can increase blood clotting and constrict blood vessels, thereby increasing the risk of heart disease, stroke and possibly cancer. Although no absolute link between omega-6 fats and breast cancer has

Reduce Consumption of Oils with Omega-6 Fat

- Corn oil
- Safflower oil
- Sunflower oil
- Peanut oil
- Cottonseed oil
- Grape seed oil
- Sesame oil

been proved, some research shows that women with breast cancer have a higher consumption of bad fats. The western diet contains up to twenty times more omega-6 as omega-3 fats; the ratio should be closer to 4:1. The American Institute for Cancer Research recommends reducing consumption of omega-6 fats.

In short, women interested in breast cancer prevention want to reduce consumption of the harmful fats found in vegetable oils, margarines, and fried, processed, or fast foods. Read labels before you buy packaged foods. Avoid products that contain hydrogenated or partially hydrogenated oils. Many diet foods or processed foods are loaded with these kinds of harmful fats.

Recommended Beverages

Good hydration is an essential to every cell in your body. It's especially important to drink a lot of water when you are undergoing chemotherapy or radiation therapy. When you drink plenty of liquids, you help flush waste and toxins from your body. Diluted fruit juice and herbal teas are also hydrating. Try to drink eight to ten eight-ounce glasses of hydrating liquids a day.

Beverages that Dehydrate

Surprisingly enough, there are some beverages that actually contribute to dehydration rather than helping to restore fluids to your system. Drinks that contain caffeine or alcohol are diuretics. They stimulate removal of water from the body. And when you lose fluids, your body is depleted of crucial nutrients, including water-soluble vitamins (such as vitamin C) and minerals (such as calcium). As a rule of thumb, you need to drink at least two glasses of water to compensate for every cup of coffee or glass of wine you drink. If you have two cups of coffee in the morning, for instance, you should try to drink four glasses of water, too.

There's an easy way to tell if you are getting dehydrated. Look at your urine. If it's dark yellow, you probably need to get more water and other liquids in your diet. Also, poor hydration contributes to fatigue. So if you often feel tired, that may be another indication that you're not getting enough hydrating liquids during the day.

What about Black and Green Teas?

Tea has less caffeine than coffee—depending on the variety, a third or even less. Although black and green teas are slightly dehydrating, drinking tea provides health benefits. Teas contain polyphenols, which are antioxidants that protect human cells from damage. Studies suggest that high levels of polyphenols in the body can reduce the risk of heart disease, fight viruses and bacteria, and reduce the risk of cancer. So have a spot of tea, but take it without milk, since the protein in milk can potentially bind to the antioxidants and render them unavailable to the body.

What about Alcohol?

A number of studies suggest that people who consume one glass of alcohol a day have an increased risk of breast cancer. On the other hand, wine (especially red wine) contains an ingredient called resveratrol, which is considered an anti-cancer agent and reduces your risk of heart disease.

If you enjoy drinking a glass of wine with your family or friends, do so in moderation. For women, the recommendation is less than one serving of an alcoholic drink per day. A serving is defined as 5 ounces of wine, 12 ounces of regular beer, or 1.5 ounces of 80-proof distilled spirits.

As for resveratrol, there are some ways to get this cancer-fighting ingredient without drinking red wine. It is also found in red grapes and in grape juice. In fact, red wine might not be the best source of this ingredient. Once the wine bottle is opened, resveratrol evaporates within twenty-four hours.

10

Coping Emotionally

In the Chinese language, the character representing the word "crisis" is a combination of two symbols, one for danger and the other for opportunity. Many breast cancer patients would say this symbol is a fitting description of a serious illness: they are frightened, but also are given the opportunity to evaluate what is really important in life. In fact, many women describe breast cancer as both the worst thing and the best thing that ever happened to them.

For someone who has just received a cancer diagnosis, it may be impossible to imagine that this could be the "best" of anything. You are immediately confronted with emotional and physical challenges that may be greater than anything you've dealt with before. How could there possibly be anything positive in this experience? But women often find they have many positive experiences during the healing, physically and emotionally.

Getting in Touch with Self

As we slow down and focus on our lives, we can explore our own needs and desires, and connect more with others for emotional and practical support. This gives us an opportunity to deepen relationships with others while developing a better understanding of ourselves. We can create more intimate and satisfying relationships. And often, we have a chance to deepen our spirituality. A feeling of connection with a higher power, with the universe, or with nature may be awakened. In times like these we learn that the human spirit has amazing strength, resilience, and capacity to overcome suffering.

As you travel the path of recovery from cancer, you'll experience strong and contradictory emotions. You may feel hopeful one moment and scared the next. One day you're completely calm and composed, the next, you're angry—at yourself, at God, at your doctors, and even at those you love.

Each woman has her own way of coping with a difficult situation. Some have easy access to their feelings and readily express themselves. Others are more reserved and private. Some women throw themselves into the cancer experience, want to know everything, and frequently talk about it. Others avoid the subject and seek distractions.

There is no right or wrong way to cope. Your emotional recovery lies in your ability to make your own needs and feelings your top priority. There are a number of steps you can take to enhance your recovery process.

Relationships with Your Doctors

When you were first diagnosed with cancer, you may have felt like you had lost control of your body and your life. Many women find that by having a good relationship with their doctors, they feel more in control and also more committed to treatment.

If you don't have an open relationship with your doctors, you can still develop one. It's never too late to start expressing your concerns or asking questions. You may feel reluctant to ask questions. But if you can overcome that reluctance and gather as much information as possible about what lies ahead, you'll reduce your anxiety.

As you continue to see your surgeon or other doctors during the course of treatment, write down your questions and concerns as you think of them. Take the list with you when you visit doctors, therapists, or other health care professionals. Remember, there is no such thing as a silly or dumb question.

Do you find it difficult to remember what was said in discussions with your doctors? You can take notes, of course, but your mind may wander as you try to deal with the implications of what you're hearing. Ask your partner, a family member, or a friend to go along to your next visit. Afterward, the two of you can review what was said and make sure your questions were answered.

Make a List of Priorities

With surgery behind you, what do you need now and in the days ahead? Take time to decide what is really important. Make a list of the activities and responsibilities you can handle. Make another list of those that are physically and emotionally draining. How many obligations can you cancel? Which items can other people take care of? Jot down the names of friends, family members, or co-workers who can help you.

Find the time to be quiet. Cry when you need to. Don't suppress emotions of fear anger and sadness.

—Rose, 59

Every day, you need to do at least one activity that makes you feel good and gives you pleasure. What brings you joy? Think of the simple and attainable pleasures that are within reach—walking in the park, sitting on your porch watching the sunset or the night sky, scratching your dog behind the ears or playing with your cat, listening to favorite music, or relaxing in a warm bath. Each day, take some time to enjoy the activities that are most comforting and make you feel happy to be alive.

Asking for Support

Many women are used to putting other people's needs—those of children, partner, family, friends and co-workers—ahead of their own. If that describes you, then you'll probably find it difficult to ask others for help. Yet it's important to learn to ask, even if you feel awkward or guilty at first. To take care of yourself, you have to reach out to other people who can provide support.

Often loved ones, even partners, would like to help, but are not sure what to say or do. Keep in mind that they, too, may be frightened and worried. They need you to let them know *how* they can help.

It's okay to tell them what you need. For example, sometimes all you need is for someone who cares about you to *just be there*—to sit with you, to listen, to let you cry.

Or maybe you need to be touched. Having your hand held, or hugging somebody, can be very healing. The direct approach is the best. It's fine to say, "Would you hold my hand?" or "I need a hug!" Right away, the other person will stop wondering what to do next or how to help.

Healing and recovery is 50 percent treatment and 50 percent loving support.

—Helen, 60

At other times, you'll need to be cheered up or distracted. You can invite others to share a meal, a cup of tea, or a laugh. A friend or family member can accompany you on a nature walk, go with you to a worship service, sit with you in a concert, or pray with you. With a simple, direct invitation, let the other person know that you'd like companionship.

Spouses, family members, and friends can also provide practical assistance to help you conserve your energy. Some people feel more comfortable showing their support by "doing" rather than talking or listening. Ask them to help you with meals. Ask them to run errands, to care for your children, to drive you to appointments.

Be as specific as possible. If someone has offered to make a meal, for instance, let them know about your or your family's favorite foods, and express your appreciation for the offer. If others offer to help take care of the children, suggest some activities that the kids enjoy.

Setting Boundaries

Not everyone is able to give you the support and the under-standing you need in the way you need it. Some of your co-workers, friends, and even family, no matter how well meaning, might say things that make you feel worse rather than better.

When others offer advice you feel you don't need, you may need to protect yourself by setting boundaries. You might politely say, "Thank you for your interest, but I'd rather not discuss this right now." Or, "I know that you are trying to be helpful and I so appreciate that, but I would prefer to get my information and treatment recommenda-tions from my doctors." This approach will not only spare their feelings, but more importantly, spare *you* needless stress and heartache.

Though family and friends want frequent updates, how can you keep everyone advised of your progress all the time? You may start to feel overwhelmed with constant telephone calls from loved ones asking how the treatments are going and how you're feeling. There are a number of ways to handle the updates, depending on your preference. Do you like to tell as many people as possible, or would you rather be more private about your health and your feelings? The following approaches can help conserve your physical and emotional energy:

- Ask one, designated person whom you trust to keep others informed.
- Use a telephone answering machine to screen your calls. When you don't have the desire or the energy to return calls, record a message that says, "Thanks for calling. I am a little tired, so I'll probably not get back to you right away. But I would love to hear your message. Please keep it under three minutes."
- E-mails, particularly group e-mails, can be an efficient and great way to keep in touch with family and friends. If you don't enjoy e-mailing, a family member or a friend can take care of this for you.

When People Pull Away

Sometimes a close friend or relative pulls away and becomes cold and distant. In extreme cases, the person may literally disappear from your life with no clear explanation. This often comes as a shock. Such an absence may be very painful to you.

Trying to understand why people do this can be exhausting and frustrating. But it's important to remember that these people are not rejecting you personally. For whatever reason, they have personal issues that have very little to do with you. Perhaps their own fear of cancer, or other fears about personal health, create feelings they can't tolerate in themselves.

If this happens, surround yourself with those who can be truly supportive. You can decide some other time whether you want to "leave the door open" for the return of someone who has not been supportive. But right now, you need people who are dependable.

Talking to Your Children

You may be tempted to protect your children, and maybe yourself, by not telling them about your diagnosis. But children can sense when something is wrong, even when they're very young. It's better to be honest with them. Tell them the truth, simply and in a manner and language appropriate to their age level.

How do you know what is age appropriate and what they need to know? You'll find out by encouraging questions from them. When they ask, give them the information they ask for, but don't offer more until they ask again. Often, children absorb stressful information in stages. After they have time to internalize the information you've given them, they will ask more questions when they are ready.

Typically when children are feeling scared and stressed, they regress, acting more like children, more babyish, less responsible. They worry that something will happen to you and that you will go away. It will help them if they can maintain their normal routines and activities as much as possible. This helps children feel secure in the knowledge that everything is okay.

Talking to Your Mate

A diagnosis of cancer can indeed strengthen the love in a relationship. Studies consistently show that the experience of going through cancer together strengthens good marriages and relationships. The process of healing brings more intimacy to a relationship and can bring couples closer together. On the other hand, if you are in an emotionally strained relationship, it may not be able to withstand this test. Your own anger, or your partner's, may surface in unanticipated ways. In a deeply troubled marriage or an abusive relationship, cancer can be a catalyst for change, liberating you and your children to create a healthier and safer life.

Hopefully, your relationship is already a strong one, and your mate is at your side to support you through your recovery. Even then, communication is important. Your needs will have changed, and your mate may not always be readily aware of what they are. Again, it's important to ask for what you need.

It's important, too, to realize what and how your mate is able to give. For example, a mate who is the silent type, probably won't become a talker after your cancer diagnosis. Someone who is not handy with homemaking tasks may not be able to take over the cooking and the house cleaning. All the same, your partner can learn new ways to help you if you express what you need to feel safe and protected. You, in turn, can accept your partner's help graciously and without criticism. Although your partner may not load the dishwasher or do the laundry just the way you like it done, your appreciation for what is offered will likely encourage further participation.

One way to ask for support is by asking your partner to accompany you when you visit your doctors. Doctor visits are an opportunity for your partner to ask questions, as well.

If you have children, encourage your partner to spend extra time with them. This not only strengthens the relationship between your mate and the children, it also makes the children feel more secure. Their outings give you a chance for time alone, if you need it.

If you feel you're having trouble communicating with your partner, or need help coping with the changes in your life and relationship, talk to your partner about seeing a marriage counselor. Often just a few sessions can get you both on the right path of love and support.

Physical and Sexual Intimacy

Women consistently express an awareness that femininity, womanhood, and sexuality are much more than having a "perfect" body. But even so, a woman who has gone through breast surgery may feel insecure about the changes in her body.

In the beginning, you may not feel the need or be ready for sexual intimacy, but you'll probably find comfort in being touched and hugged. It's very important to let your partner know that you need that kind of warm, physical contact. Sometimes, even without noticing it, couples drift apart physically.

If you notice that you and your partner have less physical contact than you used to, make an effort to start touching again. Holding hands, asking for or giving a hug, stroking an arm or back is a powerful intimate exchange between you.

Sometimes a neck or back massage is very comforting. The intimate experience can bring pleasure to both of you. Don't hesitate to ask for a massage. To make the experience more comfortable, you can either lie on your unaffected side or sit up. Your partner can massage using lotion or oil. It doesn't have to be an energetic massage. Just a gentle backrub or neckrub can be soothing, and the touching will bring you closer emotionally, as well.

Resuming Sexual Relations

If you and your partner had a rich sex life before your surgery, try to resume it again as soon as possible. Making love is life affirming. It gives you pleasure, and brings you closer together.

You may find that both you and your partner have less interest in sex than you did before your diagnosis. This is quite common. The stress of diagnosis, surgery, and possible treatment, along with the many strong emotions you're probably feeling, may reduce sexual desire.

If so, it's important to talk about those feelings. If you don't discuss those feelings there is the potential for misunderstanding and hurt feelings. But, as with all other aspects of your emotional recovery, it's important for you to be honest with yourself about your needs, concerns, and fears. Talk with your partner about them. It may help if you can start these conversations.

> *Join a support group as soon as possible. It is a great source of information and support.*
>
> —Diane, 58

Physical Comfort and Sexual Intimacy

Sometimes, partners assume that you shouldn't have sex for some time after surgery. The fear that lovemaking will hurt you may make your partner hesitant. Women often misinterpret this as rejection. You can prevent this potential misunderstanding by talking frankly. Reassure your partner that lovemaking won't harm your incisions and that it isn't bad for your health. Your partner can reassure you that you are still loved and desired.

Whenever you and your partner feel ready to have sexual relations, here are some suggestions:

- Wear something that makes you feel comfortable and desirable.
- Encourage your partner to touch your incisions. Those areas may be tender, numb, or particularly sensitive to touch, and your partner needs to be aware of that. It's important to let your partner know what feels good and what doesn't.
- Remember, there is no right or wrong position for having sex. Whatever position is comfortable for you is right.
- Protect your incision if you need to do so to relax. If so, try lying on your back with your unaffected arm crossed protectively over your treated breast and your hand resting on your affected shoulder. Alternatively, you can place a small pillow under your arm, and over your breast. If you feel safer this way, it will be easier to enjoy sex.

To make intercourse more comfortable, you can select from a number of good, nonprescription products that provide vaginal lubrication. Tamoxifen or chemotherapy can cause vaginal dryness, which makes intercourse uncomfortable.

Single Women and Sexual Intimacy

If you are a single woman without a partner, you may have some special concerns about emotional and physical intimacy. You may worry about dating and starting a new romantic relationship. You may also have concerns about when and how to tell a new friend or potential lover that you have had breast surgery.

Most single women find it can be helpful to talk to other single women who have had breast cancer. A breast cancer support group is a good place to find out how they've coped. Ask your hospital social worker, doctors, nurses—and look in the Resource section of this book—for groups that can put you in touch with other single women who have had a lumpectomy.

Overcoming Depression

It is perfectly normal to feel sad and to cry. You'll probably feel better after a good cry. However, if you feel sad all the time, you may be suffering from clinical depression.

Clinical depression is a label for a range of symptoms that are quite common, particularly among people who have experienced serious illness. An estimated 23 percent of breast cancer patients suffer from clinical depression after surgery. Receiving proper treatment, often with a combination of counseling and medications, can help one feel much better.

There are compelling reasons to treat clinical depression. Left untreated, it can interfere with physical and emotional recovery. But how do you know the difference between sadness and depression?

If you are feeling several of the following symptoms for more than two weeks, you may have clinical depression. Ask yourself, "Does this describe the way I've been feeling recently?"

- Constant and excessive feelings of worthlessness, hopelessness, guilt, shame and/or fear
- Disinterest in food, or excessive eating
- Inability to sleep, or sleeping too much
- Constant jitters or nervousness
- Not feeling pleasure; losing interest in things that used to interest you
- A loss of libido (losing interest in sex)
- Suicidal thoughts

If it seems as if you're having a lot of these symptoms, start by seeing a mental health professional who can evaluate your state of mind and recommend treatment. In addition to individual counseling with a therapist (usually a psychiatrist, psychologist, or clinical social worker), your treatment might include a combination of the following:

- Exercise
- Stress reduction techniques
- Spiritual counseling
- A support group
- Medications

Should You Take Antidepressants?

Being depressed changes your brain chemistry and sometimes the best thing you can do is to take medication. Studies have shown that only two percent of cancer patients who suffer from depression receive medication. Probably many more could be helped. Talking with a psychiatrist, a medical doctor who specializes in mental health and medications can help you.

Do something that brings you joy each day.

—Wende, 62
art therapist
breast cancer survivor

Many women who resist taking antidepressants seem to believe that the medication will make them feel happy all the time. That leads to the fear that the medication will have a dulling effect, and they won't be able to deal with sad and painful feelings. This concern is unwarranted. Antidepressants don't make you feel instantly happy, buoyant, or elated. Rather, they diminish your depression, so that you actually are better able to deal with your feelings. None of them create the feelings of euphoria that people get from recreational drugs.

How Antidepressants Work

Since depression is associated with a chemical imbalance in the brain, antidepressants come to the rescue by fine-tuning brain chemistry. The messengers that carry signals from one brain cell to another are called neurotransmitters. When neurotransmitters are out of balance, there's a risk of depression.

Commonly prescribed antidepressants include:

- Lexapro (escitalopram oxalate)
- Paxil (paroxetine)
- Prozac (fluoxetine)
- Zoloft (sertraline)
- Celexa (citalopram)
- Effexor (venlafaxine)
- Serzone (nefazadone)
- Remeron (mirtazapine)
- Wellbutrin (bupropion)

Antidepressants have side effects; some more than others. These include headache, anxiety, flushing, difficulty falling asleep, feeling jittery, problems with sexual functioning, loss of appetite, upset stomach, dizziness, and tremors. If you have problems with these or any medication, let your doctor know. The side effects may diminish as you adjust to the medications, or your psychiatrist might recommend switching to another medication that wouldn't affect you the same way.

Keep in mind that it often takes two to four weeks before antidepressants deliver their full therapeutic benefits.

Join a Support Group

After cancer surgery, you may feel different, isolated, and alone. A support group offers understanding, strength, and companionship. Surprisingly enough, you'll find humor, too—moments of belly-splitting laughter. It's such a relief to discover that you are not alone.

When you hear other women expressing feelings similar to yours, you realize that those feeling are normal and part of the healing process. In a support group, you have a safe place to express feelings that you can't or won't share with family or friends. Whether or not you have a family, your breast cancer support group becomes a family of special friends.

Before attending a meeting, call the group leader. By getting to know one person before you go, you'll feel more comfortable when you first attend. If you're not sure whether you really want to join a particular group, be sure to attend at least two meetings before you decide. Each support group has its own personality, uniquely defined by the women who participate and by the facilitator, and it takes a while to decide whether the group you visit will be a good fit. If, after a couple of meetings, you decide the group doesn't feel right, don't be discouraged. Just try another one. It's worth it. Many women say that finding a comfortable support group, and staying with it, has been vital in their emotional recovery.

Another alternative is to get in touch with another woman who has had a lumpectomy. Although her experience will not be exactly the same as yours, there is much you can share in one-on-one conversations.

Seek Spiritual Support

Spirituality and prayer can be a great source of comfort, strength, and healing. But for some women, a diagnosis of cancer marks the beginning of a spiritual crisis. Even if you have a strong spiritual life, you may begin to question everything you believe in. Feelings of betrayal are common: "Why is God punishing me?" For someone who has held to a strong faith all her life, spiritual alienation can be hard to bear.

If you have previously found comfort in spirituality, you may be ashamed about your doubts. There is no reason to hide these feelings. They are common. But don't give up on trying to find spiritual guidance. A spiritual counselor will understand your distress and, even if you feel shaken in your faith, might help you regain your spiritual balance.

Some women find their spirituality is reawakened. They may start to rethink their values, examining what is really important in life. They may rekindle relationships and develop greater intimacy. They may be inspired by acts of kindness and love.

If you are experiencing a spiritual awakening, take this opportunity to deepen it. Seek spiritual counseling, practice yoga, join a congregation, join a choir, or engage in regular prayer or meditation.

At the End of Treatment

After your surgery and any subsequent treatment is completed, you may actually feel more fragile. It's reassuring to realize that your body is healing, but your emotions may still be raw. When you finish treatment, it's particularly important to ask for and receive emotional support.

During treatment, you focus on making decisions and recovering physically. You also feel protected because you are being seen frequently by your doctors. And frankly, during treatment, most people are very sympathetic. They are compassionate when they see that you are in pain or tired. Once treatment is over and you start looking and acting like your old self, your loved ones may assume that everything is back to normal. They may become less supportive and even impatient, expecting you to get on with your life. But once you have been diagnosed with breast cancer, you know your life will never be the same.

Let the experience of breast cancer remind you to live each day to the fullest. And each day, remind yourself that you are not alone. More than two million women in the United States are living with breast cancer. These women have found, in themselves and in others, the strength and resources to recover and heal. You are part of this community of survivors.

11

Understanding Lymphedema

Lymphedema is chronic swelling caused by an accumulation of lymph fluid in the tissues, which can result when lymph nodes are removed. In the case of breast cancer surgery, several lymph nodes are often removed from the underarm area. As a result, patients are at risk for lymphedema in the affected arm, hand, or fingers.

You are at risk for lymphedema if you:

- have had multiple axillary lymph nodes removed from under your arm.
- have had radiation therapy in your underarm area and/or neck.
- are diabetic.
- get very little exercise.
- are overweight.

How the Lymph System Works

To better understand lymphedema, let's first examine the body's lymph system. The system—made up of lymph vessels, capillaries, and nodes—moves lymph fluid throughout your body. The lymph system has two main functions. First, as part of your immune system, lymph fluid carries the white blood cells that fight infection. Second, the lymph system helps remove excess fluids that naturally collect at an injury or surgery site. These fluids cause swelling, also called *edema,* which gradually subsides as the lymph drainage system carries away the excess fluid.

How Lymphedema Develops

When lymph nodes are removed, your lymphatic system is easily overloaded. It is no longer as capable of carrying away the extra fluid in the tissues of your affected hand and arm. That is why you are susceptible to the chronic swelling that characterizes lymphedema. Lymphedema may occur soon after surgery, or it can occur anytime over the course of one's life. Some women have developed lymphedema as long as twenty years after surgery.

Why Lymph Nodes Are Removed

During breast cancer surgery, a surgeon may remove several lymph nodes from the underarm area, called the *axilla*, to test them for the presence of cancer cells. If cancer cells are found, it's an indication that the cancer has spread outside the breast. In performing axillary lymph node sampling, a surgeon typically removes between seven and fourteen lymph nodes of the thirty-five or so in that area. (The body has about 800 lymph nodes.)

Whether or not cancer cells are found in the lymph nodes, removing them creates a risk for developing lymphedema. The more lymph nodes removed, the higher the risk of developing lymphedema.

Fortunately, the new procedure to test lymph nodes, sentinel node biopsy, involves removing only one or two lymph nodes. This surgical advancement places women at minimal risk.

Learn about lymphedema. The more you know about lymphedema prevention the less likely you will develop it.

— Janice
nurse

Stages of Lymphedema

The first signs of lymphedema are often subtle, maybe only a slight swelling in one part of your affected hand or arm, maybe only on the wrist or a single finger. If you receive treatment for lymphedema in its early stages, you can prevent it from getting worse. There are three grades of lymphedema. (Note that the grades of lymphedema have no relationship to the grade of a tumor.)

Grade I

The earliest stage, Grade I or "acute lymphedema," is also referred to as "pitting edema." You can test for it by pressing on a swollen area with your finger. If you see an indentation or pit, you may have an early stage lymphedema. The swelling should go down promptly if you elevate your arm. Acute lymphedema generally responds to prompt and proper treatment. If you do not receive proper treatment, the lymphedema may progress to Grade II lymphedema, usually after three to six months.

Grade II

In Grade II, swelling on the affected side becomes more obvious. The tissue feels spongy and is non-pitting, which means when the skin is pressed with a finger, bounces back. With Grade II lymphedema, the skin also hardens as fibrous tissue develops, a condition called *fibrosis*. The hardened tissue further blocks lymph flow, which makes the lymphedema worse.

Grade III

At this stage, the swelling becomes extensive. The skin and underlying tissue become hard or fibrous. If lymphedema goes untreated, there's an added risk of an infection, *cellulitis*, which forms as a result of the stagnant excess fluid collecting in the tissues. This fluid is full of protein, which is food for bacteria.

Cellulitis: A Medical Emergency

If you have cellulitis, you may have a rash, and your skin will be slightly swollen and warm to the touch. As cellulitis progresses, you may develop one or several red lines running up your arm. Then, in only a few hours, a large area or the whole arm may become very red, swollen, hot, and quite painful. These infection symptoms indicate full-blown cellulitis. At this point you may also feel tired and unwell, and you may have a fever.

As soon as you see any symptoms of cellulitis, seek medical attention immediately. You will need appropriate antibiotic therapy, which usually starts with oral antibiotics, followed by IV therapy if the condition worsens. Without treatment, cellulitis can lead to septic shock (blood poisoning) and eventual death.

A small wound, particularly if it's properly treated, rarely develops into cellulitis. But if any cut or sore becomes infected and you let it go, there is a real danger of this infection turning into cellulitis. If cellulitis is developing, you can usually better detect the signs by examining your skin in natural daylight.

If you notice chronic swelling (lymphedema) make sure that you start treatment. Lymphedema can and should be treated.

—Linda
nurse

Treatment for Lymphedema

Lymphedema Therapists

Unfortunately, most medical doctors lack the specialized training to treat lymphedema. However, hundreds of certified lymphedema thera-pists are available in the United States and Canada. They include some nurses, physical and occupational therapists, and licensed massage therapists, as well as a small number of medical doctors. Contact the

National Lymphedema Network, listed in the Resources section in this book, to find a trained therapist near you.

Lymphedema Therapy Treatments

Any swelling that persists for more than three days should be evaluated, even if the swelling goes down after elevating your arm. Ideally, you should start treatment within two weeks of noticing any persistent recurring swelling.

A woman undergoing lymphedema treatment should have several treatments a week for four to eight weeks or until swelling subsides. Treatment sessions last about an hour. The most effective treatment will include the following steps:

- Education: Since the risk of lymphedema lasts a lifetime, it's important to know as much about it as possible.
- Antibiotic therapy: Before treatment can actually begin, you must be free of infection. The lymphedema therapist will evaluate you for any signs of infection and will work with a doctor to prescribe appropriate antibiotic therapy (usually penicillin).
- Cleaning and lubricating the skin.
- *Manual lymph drainage (MLD)*: With this special massage technique, the therapist uses gentle pressure to move the fluid back into the vascular system and reduce swelling.
- Bandaging and wrapping the hand and arm. After MLD is performed, the therapist wraps the hand and arm with special bandages (not Ace or elastic-type bandages). The greatest pressure is on the hand; pressure is decreased on the higher parts of the arm. The bandage stays on until the next treatment.
- Breathing and muscle-building exercises: After the bandages are applied, the therapist will have you perform several breathing and muscle contraction exercises that increase lymphatic flow and drainage.

- Compression sleeve: At the end of the course of treatments, you will be fitted with a compression sleeve. The sleeve replaces the bandages and wrapping. This sleeve is worn during the day to maintain the benefits of treatment and to prevent or slow the accumulation of fluid.
- Regular follow-up: Routine follow-up is important. You may need additional treatment on an annual basis.

Preventing Lymphedema

Because lymphedema may occur at anytime over the course of your life, it is important to develop lifelong habits to help prevent it. Many of the things you do every day can affect your risk for lymphedema. By modifying how you dress, work, exercise, and travel, you can minimize your risk. Pay special attention to the following lifestyle factors.

Avoid Tight Clothing and Jewelry

It's important to avoid wearing tight rings, watches, or bracelets that could constrict lymph flow. You also need to avoid carrying a heavy purse, handbag, or luggage with a strap that goes over your affected shoulder. And avoid any garments, such as those with tight wrist bands, which constrict flow through the arm.

Avoid Repetitive Stress Injuries

Working nonstop at any task that involves your affected hand and arm, especially if you do it for several days in a row, may lead to lymphedema. Most people are aware that working improperly at the computer is one cause of repetitive stress injury, but there are other causes as well. Tasks such as gardening, knitting, drawing, and painting may also lead to stress injuries.

To avoid these injuries, take a short break every twenty minutes and stretch your upper body, especially your hands and arms. Also, do regular, moderate exercises to strengthen your hands and arms.

Exercise

Regular, moderate exercise reduces your risk for lymphedema and infections by stimulating lymphatic flow and improving circulation. Water aerobics and swimming are excellent forms of exercise for preventing lymphedema. The water acts like a natural compression garment for your arm, and it keeps you cool, so you don't risk overheating. Being overheated may lead to dehydration, which increases the risk of lymphedema.

Be Cautious with Vigorous Exercise

If you enjoy more strenuous activities such as weight training with heavy weights, long-distance bike riding, tennis, cross-country skiing, or basketball, you need to take some specific precautions to avoid lymphedema. Why? When you exercise strenuously, the muscles in your upper body fill with blood. This can overload your lymphatic system. Similarly, injury to a muscle may cause fluid to collect.

If you notice swelling when you perform an exercise or sport, you need to consider modifying it or giving it up. But the following tips may enable you to continue exercising safely:

- Don't exercise to the point that you are sore. When muscles hurt, they are injured.
- Drink plenty of water, and don't push yourself on hot days.
- Pace yourself. Take breaks at least every twenty minutes to breathe and stretch.
- If you develop swelling during an exercise session, stop immediately.
- Wear a compression sleeve on the affected arm. This specially designed sleeve is like support hose for your arm, exerting the most pressure near your wrist. Purchase a correctly designed

sleeve. Don't make it yourself. Wear it for activities such as golf, tennis, biking, or strength training.

- Avoid very hot showers or baths, saunas, hot tubs, or steam rooms especially after a vigorous workout.

Prepare for Air Travel

Air travel, and preparing for it, increase your risk for lymphedema. This happens for several reasons. Often, you're busy before taking a trip—cleaning your home, washing, ironing, and packing. The extra activity may overload the lymphatic system. The day of the flight, you may be carrying a heavy suitcase and you may reach and strain to get your bag into the overhead bin.

During the flight, you may become dehydrated since air in the plane is very dry. And you stay seated for many hours, impeding blood flow. You may be hot and thirsty when the plane lands. That's when you may notice that your hand or arm is swollen.

You can avoid at least some of these problems if you take the following measures:

- In the days before your trip, pace yourself, and don't overuse your affected arm.
- Do not carry heavy baggage on your affected side. Ask for help placing your bag in the overhead compartment and getting it down.
- Stay well hydrated. Drink a lot of fluids and avoid alcohol or caffeinated drinks, which are dehydrating.
- Reserve a seat where your affected arm is not near the aisle, so that it won't be bumped and injured by a passenger or beverage cart.
- Every hour, move about the cabin and perform five arm pump exercises.
- Wear a compression sleeve for the entire flight.

Preventing Injury and Infection

Since the lymph system is part of your immune system, you are at greater risk of getting infections from even small cuts or wounds, and any untreated infection can lead to lymphedema. Preventing injury and infection is especially important for women who have diabetes; diabetics have a higher risk of infections since their healing ability is often impaired.

Prevent Wound Infection

If you get a scrape, scratch, or cut on your affected side, you must treat the wound appropriately, even if the wound seems quite small. To prevent getting cuts and scratches, it's a good idea to wear protective gloves and clothing for tasks that might lead to injury. These include housework, home maintenance, yard work, gardening, and baking.

If you do suffer a wound, here are the steps you should take to prevent infection:

- Vigorously wash the wound with soap and warm water for at least 20 seconds, twice a day.
- Apply a topical antibiotic to the wound. Prescription Bactroban (2% mupirocin calcium cream) is the best topical antibiotic.
- Cover the wound with a bandage or sterile gauze dressing, and keep it dry.
- Check the wound twice a day for any signs of infection: redness, swelling, warmth, pus, and increased pain.

If you take these preventive measures and still see signs of infection, you'll need oral antibiotics. If you cannot reach your doctor, go to an emergency room.

Some doctors will give you prescription antibiotics in advance if you plan to travel or if you live far away from a pharmacy. This can be very helpful if you enjoy camping or plan to travel internationally. Also, ask your doctor about topical and oral antibiotics that you can carry with you.

Prevent Fingernail Infection

The hand on your affected side requires some special attention, particularly in the area around your fingernails, which may become infected if you get a hangnail. Give yourself gentle manicures by gently pushing back your cuticles. Don't cut the cuticles, since they protect your nail from infection. Use your own manicuring tools and don't share them. Make a habit of cleaning them with rubbing alcohol.

If you enjoy having your nails done professionally, take your own manicuring tools to the manicurist. Unfortunately, many nail salons do not sterilize their instruments, so it's essential to take your own.

Avoid applying artificial nails. Toxic chemicals are used to apply them, and the chemicals tend to ruin the natural nail. This can be a source of fungal infection.

Prevent Insect Bites

Some women develop large welts when bitten by insects. Such injuries may lead to lymphedema. The best measure is prevention. Wear long-sleeved shirts and apply insect repellent liberally. If you do get bitten, here's what to do:

- Take an antihistamine (such as Benadryl), which will help reduce swelling. (Be aware that Benadryl can make you feel drowsy.)
- Take an anti-inflammatory drug such as ibuprofen (Advil).
- Apply topical cortisone cream to reduce inflammation.
- Apply an ice compress, twenty minutes on and ten minutes off.

With treatment, any welt caused by an insect bite should resolve in an hour or so. If it doesn't, you should call your doctor.

Prevent Skin Irritation

Your skin acts as a barrier that keeps bacteria and viruses from entering your body, but this protection may be impaired if your skin is dry and cracked. To keep your skin pliant, always use a mild soap, such as Cetaphil, Basis, and unscented Dove, particularly on your affected hand and arm. After you bathe, vigorously but gently rub your skin with a towel to remove dry and dead skin. Then apply a lotion. Eucerine is especially good because it lowers the pH level (thereby increasing the acidity) of your skin. A lower pH inhibits bacteria growth.

When you shave under your arm, you may accidentally cut the skin, particularly if that area is numb to the touch. If you must shave, use an electric razor rather than a straight-edge razor.

It's also important to prevent sunburn. Wear protective clothing or use a generous amount of sunscreen when you're going to be outdoors for any length of time.

12

Follow-up Care

You've made it through a breast cancer diagnosis. You've made it through breast surgery, radiation, and perhaps chemotherapy and hormonal therapy. In many respects, things are getting back to normal. Still, things will never be quite the same: in the back of your mind is the scary thought that breast cancer can recur. Virtually every woman who has had breast cancer copes with these thoughts. Remember, most women survive breast cancer and live long lives.

Be reassured by the fact that you'll be carefully monitored by your doctors with regular follow-up care. If no health problems arise, doctors usually like to see patients every three to six months for the first five years, and then twice yearly thereafter.

You may be seeing several doctors—your surgeon, medical oncologist, radiation oncologist, as well as your regular internist or gynecologist. You may be tempted to make all your appointments in the same month. However, by spacing out your appointments, your doctors will be able to monitor you more closely. To help keep on top of all your appointments, make your next appointment before you leave your doctor's office.

Keeping a Symptom Journal

It may be reassuring to know that a symptom that comes and then goes away is *not* a sign of cancer recurrence. However, a symptom that persists and worsens over time can be a sign of recurrence.

You can help your doctors by noting any subtle changes in your body since the last visit. Some women find that it's helpful to keep a symptom journal. If you notice a new symptom, describe it and note the date it started. If the symptom causes discomfort, grade the severity of the discomfort, using a scale from 1 (mild) to 10 (severe pain). With such a record, you'll see a pattern of any symptoms.

If you've having any pain or any persistent and worsening symptom that lasts for more than one week, don't wait until your next scheduled follow-up visit. Make an appointment to see your surgeon or medical oncologist as soon as possible. If you put off seeing your doctor, you may constantly worry about a recurrence. However, if you go in, you'll most likely find out that you are okay.

Most women will survive breast cancer and live long lives.

—Mark R.
radiation oncologist

Follow-up Visits to Your Surgeon

Your surgeon is the best doctor to give you a thorough breast examination. And your surgeon is the doctor to exam you if you have any concerns regarding a new lump or change in the appearance of your breasts.

Your surgeon will be watchful of any signs of cancer at the lumpectomy scar, the most common site of local recurrence. Your doctor will also carefully check your unaffected breast. Signs of local recurrence are:

- a new lump or thickening
- a rash that does not go away
- an enlarged, non-tender lymph node in the armpit or above the collar bone

Your surgeon will also order yearly mammograms of both breasts. Some surgeons recommended twice-yearly mammograms of the treated breast. If your breast tissue is especially dense, a yearly breast MRI may be helpful.

Follow-up Visits to Your Oncologist

During your regularly scheduled visit, your medical oncologist will take a careful history, perform a physical exam, and when appropriate, order tests. Medical oncologists monitor for signs and symptoms that cancer has recurred in the body, that is, metastatic disease.

The oncologist needs your help to detect symptoms that may be of concern. If you report any persistent and worsening symptoms, your doctor may then decide to have tests done. Since you and the doctor are working hand in hand to monitor your health, you need to be aware of symptoms of metastatic disease so that you can report them immediately. The most common sites of breast cancer metastasis, in order of prevalence, are bone, lung, liver, and brain.

Symptoms of Cancer Recurrence

Bone Metastasis

A localized pain that hurts continually may be a sign of a tumor growing within the bone. The pain may not necessarily feel like it is coming from the bone, but it is constant—it usually remains at night and it does not improve with time.

Certainly, if you suffer from arthritis you may have constant joint pain.

So if you report this kind of pain, the medical oncologist will usually order an X-ray or bone scan to distinguish between arthritis and bone metastasis. A *bone scan* is a diagnostic test in which a small amount of radioactive substance is injected into the bloodstream. By tracing the radioactive substance, a scanner can detect any areas of increased blood circulation in the bone, indicating the presence of cancer.

Lung Metastasis

Usually a tumor in the lung does not cause pain. However, if a tumor takes up space in a major airway, it might cause wheezing or shortness of breath and a constant, dry cough. These symptoms typically get worse; the common cold or flu, on the other hand, gets better. A medical oncologist may use chest X-rays to make a diagnosis.

Liver Metastasis

Symptoms of a liver metastasis result from a tumor taking up space in the liver and impeding its function. Symptoms may be subtle at first, but may include unexplained and worsening fatigue, weight loss, loss of appetite, and nausea. Cancer in the liver may also cause discomfort in the right abdomen, above where the liver is located.

The first test a doctor is likely to order is a simple blood test that will reveal whether liver enzymes are elevated. If so, an oncologist will probably request a CT scan or ultrasound scan of the liver. A CT scan, a computer-aided X-ray, shows three-dimensional images of the liver. Ultrasound testing uses high-frequency sound waves to check the liver.

Brain Metastasis

One symptom of a brain tumor is a constant or recurring headache. But, of course, many women get tension headaches that have nothing whatever to do with a tumor. The difference is that a headache associated with brain metastasis typically begins in the morning, before one gets out of bed, but then improves as the day goes on. This is different from a tension headache, which usually starts during the day and gradually gets worse. Be sure to tell your doctor about any recurring headaches and try to describe them as thoroughly as possible.

There are other possible symptoms. Sometimes drowsiness, nausea, or both accompany these headaches. Some patients have seizures. Other symptoms may be similar to those of a stroke—an inability to walk, weakness in parts of the body, or vision problems.

To make an accurate diagnosis, oncologists rely on a CT scan or an magnetic resonance imaging (*MRI*), a diagnostic test that uses a powerful magnet and radio waves to show the number of blood vessels in tissue. Since cancers have more blood vessels than healthy tissue, brain tumors show up as distinct images in a CT scan or MRI.

Can Recurrence Be Detected Early?

Currently, doctors are able to determine whether cancer has recurred only when symptoms are observable. Unfortunately, there are few tools to help doctors detect metastasis before a tumor starts to grow. Frequent scans, such as CT scans, could be done, but scans are not capable of detecting a *micrometastasis*, the microscopic spread of cancerous cells to other organs. And micrometastasis may remain dormant for many years or your whole life.

> *You are on a journey.*
> *Treat yourself gently and*
> *expect the best of your family*
> *and friends.*
>
> —Carol, 55
> psychologist
> breast cancer survivor

However, some medical oncologists perform routine blood tests to detect antigens, substances that some breast cancer tumors shed into the bloodstream. Also known as *tumor markers*, these substances *may* signal the presence of cancer in the body. If tumor marker levels decrease after chemotherapy or hormonal treatment, it indicates a good response to treatment. If tumor marker levels increase it may be a sign of resistance to treatment or a recurrence. Three tumor marker tests commonly used to detect breast cancer are Cancer Antigen 15-3 (CA15-3), Cancer Antigen 27.29 (CA27.29) and Carcinoembryonic Antigen (CEA).

Still, these tests are controversial because they are not very sensitive or specific. They are not sensitive enough to detect very early recurrence, since a tumor must be large enough to release tumor markers in detectable amounts. Also, these tests may yield false positives, indicating a positive or abnormal result when, in fact, no abnormal condition exists.

Performing Monthly Breast Self-Examinations

You are encouraged to do your own *breast self-examination (BSE)* every month. After breast surgery, many women find this scary, but, by learning how to examine yourself, you may feel more in control and less fearful. Breast self-examination will allow you to detect any changes that may be of concern, such as a lump, a visible change, swelling or infection.

During this visual exam, notice whether you have any of the following changes and tell your surgeon about them:

- persistent rash or a red area on your scar, chest, or breast
- persistent itchy rash on your nipple or areola
- nipple discharge that is spontaneous and persistent
- a change in the size or shape of your breast, such as a dimple
- any lump in your breast, chest, scar, or underarm area
- swelling or signs of cellulitis in your arm

Ask your doctor or nurse to show you how to do a BSE, or check with your local hospital to find a nurse who can teach you.

Resources

Breast Cancer Action

55 New Montgomery St., Suite 624
San Francisco, California 94105
1-415-243-9301
www.bcaction.org

An activist and advocacy organization of breast cancer survivors
and their supporters; its purpose is to increase the awareness of
breast cancer among those in government, the scientific
community, private industry, and the media. The organization
publishes a newsletter.

The Susan G. Komen Breast Cancer Foundation

5005 LBJ Freeway
Suite 250
Dallas, TX 75244
Phone: 972-855-600
www.komen.org
www.breastcancerinfo.com

A nonprofit organization with a network of volunteers in local
chapters throughout the United States, this foundation organizes
the *Race for the Cure* events in cities across the United States. Its
mission is to eradicate breast cancer as a life-threatening disease by
advancing research, education, screening, and treatment.

National Coalition for Cancer Survivorship (NCCS)
1010 Wayne Avenue
Suite 770
Silver Spring, MD 20910-5600
Phone: 301-650-9127 or 877 NCCS-YES (877-622-7937)
www. cancersearch.org

Founded in 1986 by and for people with cancer and those who care for them, NCCS is a patient-led advocacy organization working on behalf of people with all types of cancer and their families. Its mission is to ensure quality cancer care for all Americans by leading and strengthening the survivorship movement, empowering cancer survivors, and advocating for policy issues that affect cancer survivors' quality of life.

The Breast Cancer Fund (TBCF)
2107 O'Farrell Street
San Francisco, CA 94115
Phone: 415-346-8223
www.breastcancerfund.org

TBCF (or "The Fund") is a nonprofit organization formed in 1992 to innovate and accelerate the response to the breast cancer crisis. The mission of The Fund is to end breast cancer and to make sure the best medical care, support services, and information are available to all women.

National Alliance of Breast Cancer Organizations (NABCO)
9 East 37th Street, 10th Floor
New York, NY 10016
Phone: 888-80-NABCO, or 888-806-2226
www.nabco.org

NABCO is a nonprofit organization offering information and educational resources on breast cancer. NABCO provides information to medical professionals, patients and their families. It advocates beneficial regulatory change and legislation.

Celebrating Life Foundation (CLF)

P.O. Box 224076
Dallas, TX 75222-4076
Phone: 800-207-0992
www.celebratinglife.org

This nonprofit organization is devoted to educating the African-American community and women of color about the risk of breast cancer. CLF encourages advancements in the early detection and treatment among these women, and works for the improvement of survival rates.

American Cancer Society (ACS)

15999 Clifton Rd NE
Atlanta, GA 30329-4251
Phone: 800-ACS-2345 (800-227-2345)
www.cancer.org

A national, nonprofit organization with local chapters that provides education, emotional and practical support programs. The ACS "Reach for Recovery" program provides one-to-one emotional support and information by trained volunteers who are breast cancer survivors. "Look Good. Feel Better." is a free workshop for women undergoing treatment for cancer. The workshop covers using turbans, scarves, wigs, and makeup. The ACS web site offers news and health information about the nature of breast cancer and its causes, risk factors, and treatment. The site also features message boards and chat rooms.

Cancer Care, Inc.

275 7th Ave.
New York, NY 10001
Phone: 212-302-2400 (800-813-HOPE)
www.cancercare.org

A nonprofit organization since 1994, Cancer Care offers emotional support, information, and practical help to people with all types of cancer and their loved ones. All services are free. Oncology social workers are available for phone consultations in which they provide emotional counseling and support. Cancer Care also offers education seminars, teleconferences, and referrals to other services.

Y-Me National Breast Cancer Organization

212 W. Van Buren, Suite 500
Chicago, IL 60607
Phone: 312-986-8338
24-hour Y-ME National Breast Cancer Hotlines:
800-221-2141 English
800-986-9505 Spanish
www.Y-ME.org

In addition to its advocacy role, Y-Me provides information, peer support, and referral. Y-Me has chapters throughout the country that offer support groups, and its web site is available in Spanish as well as English. Callers can talk with trained volunteers who are breast cancer survivors.

AMC Cancer Research Center & Foundation

1600 Pierce Street
Denver, CO 80214
Phone: 303-233-6501
800-321-1557

800-535-3777 Cancer Information and Counseling Line
www.amc.org

This not-for-profit research institute is dedicated to the prevention of cancer and other chronic diseases. AMC conducts cancer research in the areas of causation and prevention. Its other areas of research are nutrition (for the prevention of disease), health communications, behavioral research, and community studies.

The National Lymphedema Network (NLN)

Latham Square, 1611 Telegraph Avenue, Suite 1111
Oakland, CA 94612-2138
Tel: 510-208-3200
Fax: 510-208-3110
Infoline: 1-800-541-3259
www.lymphnet.org

The NLN provides education for the prevention and treatment of lymphedema. Its hotline offers support, information, and referrals for treatment of lymphedema. The NLN publishes a quarterly newsletter.

The Cancer Information Service (CIS)

National Institutes of Health
Bethesda, MD 20892-2580
Phone: 301-496-4000
1-800-4-CANCER (800-422-6237)
www.cancernet.nci.nih.gov

The National Cancer Institute is part of the National Institutes of Health and is the federal government's principal agency for cancer research and control. The CIS offers free written material and information about treatment, support services, medical facilities, second opinion centers, and clinical trials. Trained information specialists answer cancer-related questions.

OncoLink

The University of Pennsylvania Medical Center
3400 Spruce Street – 2 Donner
Philadelphia, PA 19104
www.oncolink.upenn.edu/disease/breast

Maintained by the University of Pennsylvania, OncoLink's mission is to help cancer patients, families, health-care professionals, and the general public receive accurate cancer-related information at no charge. OncoLink offers comprehensive information about specific types of cancer, updates on cancer treatments, and news about research advances. The information (updated every day) is provided at various levels, from introductory to in-depth.

The U.S. National Library of Medicine

8600 Rockville Pike
Bethesda, MD 20894
www.nlm.nih.gov
MEDLINEplus www.nlm.nih.gov/medlineplus

Produced by the National Library of Medicine, this site indexes articles from more than 3,500 medical journals. The service is aimed primarily at scientists and health professionals; however, MEDLINEplus is written for consumers.

Glossary

A

adjuvant therapy: Treatment added to increase the effectiveness of primary therapy; chemotherapy, hormonal therapy, and radiation therapy. Usually given after surgery to prevent or delay recurrence. Neoadjuvant therapy is given before surgery, usually to shrink the tumor.

aneuploid: Cells containing abnormal amounts of DNA. Aneuploid tumors are fast growing.

areola: Area of pigmentation around the nipple.

axilla: Armpit.

axillary lymph nodes: Lymph nodes located in the armpit area. Breast cancer cells can travel to the axillary lymph nodes. One of these, called sentinel node, or a number of them may be removed to test for the presence of cancer cells.

axillary lymph node sampling: Surgical removal of some of the lymph nodes found in the armpit region.

B

bilateral: Involving both sides, as in a bilateral mastectomy.

blood count: Blood test to measure the number of red blood cells, white blood cells, and platelets.

bone marrow: The soft inner part of large bones that produces red blood cells, white blood cells, and platelets.

bone scan: Test to determine the presence of cancer in the bones.

BRCA1 and BRCA2: Mutated genes associated with hereditary breast and ovarian cancer. May be inherited from father's or mother's side of the family. About 10 percent of breast cancers are inherited.

breast reconstruction: Surgical creation of the breast contour, nipple, and areola. Performed by a plastic surgeon.

breast self-examination (BSE): Examination of the breast, chest, and lymph nodes by a woman herself.

C

cancer: General term for more than one hundred diseases characterized by the abnormal and uncontrolled growth of cells. Also called *malignancy.*

carcinogen: Substance that can cause cancer.

carcinoma: Cancers that arise from the skin, the lining of internal organs, and glands. Breast carcinoma arises from the milk-producing glands and/or ducts.

CT scan (Computer tomography): A study that creates three-dimensional images of organs and structures inside the body. Used to detect the presence of cancer in the major organs in the body.

cell: The smallest structural unit of living tissue that can survive and reproduce on its own.

cellulitis: Infection of soft tissue. The tissue quickly becomes red, hot, swollen, and painful.

chemotherapy: Cancer treatment using cytotoxic (cell-killing) drugs. Chemotherapy is administered when there is the risk that cancer cells have spread.

clinical breast examination: Examination of the breast, chest, and lymph nodes performed by a health care provider. The examination consists of a visual and a touch (palpation) examination.

cytotoxic: Causing the death of cells. The term usually refers to drugs used in chemotherapy.

D

DCIS (ductal carcinoma in situ): The earliest stage of breast cancer in which abnormal cells remain in the ducts and have not invaded (infiltrated) the surrounding tissue. DCIS is also referred to as *intraductal cancer.*

differentiated: Clearly defined. Well-differentiated cells closely resemble normal cells and are slow growing. Poorly differentiated cells look very different from normal cells and are fast growing.

144

diploid: Cells containing normal amounts of DNA. Diploid tumors are slow growing.

DNA (deoxyribonucleic acid): The genetic material contained in the nucleus of the cell. The DNA of cancer cells is analyzed to see whether they have the normal amount of DNA (diploid) or an abnormal amount (aneuploid).

drain: Tube inserted during surgery to drain fluids that accumulate after surgery.

ducts: Channels in the breast that carry milk to the nipple.

E

edema: Swelling caused by a collection of fluid in the soft tissue.

estrogen: Female sex hormones produced by the ovaries, adrenal glands, placenta, and fat. There are three types: estriol, estradiol, and estrone.

estrogen receptor: Protein found on some cells to which other molecules such as estrogen and progesterone will attach. If a breast cancer tumor tests positive for estrogen receptors, it is sensitive to estrogen.

F

flap: A portion of the latissimus dorsi muscle, along with fat, and skin and its blood supply, that is moved to the chest to reconstruct a breast.

G

gene: The basic unit of heredity. Each gene is composed of DNA and occupies a certain location on a chromosome, a linear thread in the nucleus of a cell. DNA, genes, and chromosomes together or individually are referred to as "genetic material."

genetic: Relating to genes or inherited characteristics.

grading: Classification of cancers according to the appearance of cancer cells under the microscope. Low-grade cancer grows more slowly than high-grade cancer.

H

hematoma: A mass of blood that can form in a wound after surgery or trauma.

Her2: An oncogene that when overexpressed, leads to more cell growth. Also called erb-B2.

hormone: Chemical substance produced by a gland or a number of glands. There are many kinds of hormones, which act like chemical messengers. They enter the bloodstream and cause effects in other tissues.

hormone receptor test: Diagnostic test to determine whether a breast cancer's growth is influenced by hormones (estrogen or progesterone) and, therefore, whether it can be treated with hormonal therapy.

hot flashes: Sensation of heat and/or flushing that occurs suddenly. This and other menopausal symptoms may be a side effect of chemotherapy and hormonal therapy.

hysterectomy: Surgical procedure in which the uterus is removed.

I

immune system: The body's system for promoting healing and killing viruses, bacteria, and cancer cells.

inflammatory breast cancer: A particularly aggressive form of breast cancer that is usually treated with chemotherapy first, and then with a mastectomy and radiation therapy.

invasive cancer: Breast cancer that has broken out of the milk ducts and/or lobules and infiltrated surrounding tissue. Invading does not imply that the cancer is fast growing or that it has spread outside the breast. Also called infiltrating.

L

LCIS (lobular carcinoma in situ): Atypical lobular cells. The presence of LCIS indicates a higher risk for developing either invasive lobular or invasive ductal cancer in either breast.

linear accelerator: The machine most commonly used to deliver radiation therapy.

lobule: The part of the breast that produces and stores milk.

lumpectomy: Surgical procedure that removes the cancer and the surrounding rim of healthy tissue. This breast conservation procedure is usually followed by six to seven weeks of radiation therapy to the breast.

lymphedema: Chronic swelling of the hand and/or arm. This condition is a possible lifelong complication from removing the axillary lymph nodes or treating them with radiation therapy.

lymph nodes: Small, bean-shaped glands found throughout the body that help eliminate bacteria, viruses, and cancer cells.

M

malignant: Cancerous.

mastectomy: Surgical removal of the breast. A modified radical mastectomy removes the breast and some of the lymph nodes under the arm. A simple mastectomy removes only the breast.

metastasis: Spread of breast cancer cells to another organ, such as the bones, lungs, liver, or brain.

micrometastasis: Microscopic and as yet undetectable but presumed spread of cancerous cells to other organs.

MRI (magnetic resonance imaging): Diagnostic test that uses a powerful magnet and radio waves to detect cancer in different organs in the body.

mutation: An alteration in the structure of a gene.

N

nadir: The lowest point in a patient's blood count, usually seven to ten days after a chemotherapy treatment.

negative lymph nodes: Lymph nodes that are free of cancer cells.

neoadjuvant therapy: Chemotherapy or hormonal therapy given before surgery usually to shrink the tumor.

nucleus: The central body of a cell that regulates cell growth, metabolism and reproduction, and transmits characteristics of the cell when it divides.

O

oncologist: Doctor who specializes in the treatment of cancer. A radiation oncologist specializes in the treatment of cancer with radiation therapy; a medical oncologist specializes in treatment with medication; and a surgical oncologist specializes in treatment with surgery.

oncology: The study of cancer.

oncology nurse: Nurse who specializes in the care and recovery of patients with cancer. She or he is a good resource for symptom management, educational material, and information on emotional support.

P

palpation: Examination by touch.

pathologist: Doctor who specializes in examining tissue under a microscope and diagnosing disease.

pathology report: Report of the analysis and tests performed on tissue removed in surgery.

pectoralis major and minor: Major muscles that lie under the breast and over the rib cage.

plastic surgeon: Doctor who specializes in surgically creating a breast contour, nipple, and areola.

platelets: Cells in the blood necessary for clotting to help the body stop bleeding.

positive: Cancer cells are present.

progesterone: A female hormone.

R

radiologist: Doctor who interprets imaging studies such as mammograms, MRIs, bone scans, and CT scans, to diagnose disease.

recurrence: Return of a cancer after the initial treatment. Local recurrence occurs at the original tumor site.

red blood cells (RBC): Also called erythrocytes, these cells give blood its color. These cells carry oxygen from the lungs throughout the body.

retraction: A drawing-in of the nipple or the skin of breast, which can be a sign of breast cancer.

S

S-phase fraction: Measurement of how many cells are dividing at a given time. A low S-phase indicates a slow-growing tumor; a high S-phase indicates a fast-growing tumor.

sentinel node: The first lymph node that drains from the tumor; therefore, the first node in which spreading cancer cells are likely to show up.

sentinel node biopsy: Surgical procedure that removes the sentinel node for examination under a microscope. If the sentinel node is free of cancer, the other axillary nodes need not be removed and examined, so that pain, nerve damage, and the risk of lymphedema are minimized.

systemic treatment: Treatment of the whole body, such as chemotherapy and/or hormonal therapy.

T

tamoxifen (Nolvadex): Oral medication commonly used as hormonal therapy for estrogen receptor positive tumors. Has been used and studied for twenty years, and has been demonstrated to reduce the rate of recurrence.

toxic: Poisonous.

tumor: Abnormal mass of tissue.

U

ultrasound (sonogram): Test that uses high-frequency sound waves to generate images of internal organs or tumors. An ultrasound can determine whether a lump is a benign, fluid-filled cyst or whether it is solid.

W

white blood cells (WBC): Also called leukocytes, these cells are part of the body's defense against infection.

Index

About the Authors

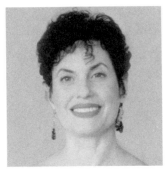

Rosalind Benedet, R.N., M.S.N., N.P., is the director of the Breast Cancer Recovery Program at the California Pacific Medical Center's Breast Health Center in San Francisco. A certified nurse practitioner in women's health, Ms. Benedet received her nursing degree and her master's in nursing science at the Massachusetts General Hospital Institute of Health Professionals in Boston. She is a native of San Francisco.

Ms. Benedet is also the author of *After Mastectomy—Healing Physically and Emotionally* (Addicus Books, 2003).

Mark C. Rounsaville, M.D., is a radiation oncologist in practice at California Pacific Medical Center in San Francisco. After graduating from Auburn University in Auburn, Alabama, Dr. Rounsaville attended the University of South Florida College of Medicine in Tampa. He received board certification in radiation oncology from the American Board of Radiology. Dr. Rounsaville is a member of several professional organizations, including the California Medical Association, American Society of Therapeutic Radiologists and Oncologists, American Society of Clinical Oncology, Northern California Radiation Oncology Society, and American Society of Breast Disease.

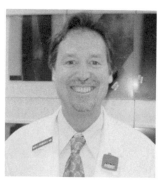

Dr. Rounsaville is the author of numerous scientific journal articles and is an assistant clinical professor of radiation oncology at the University of California San Francisco School of Medicine.

Also from Addicus Books

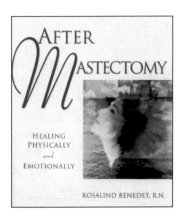

After Mastectomy
Healing Physically & Emotionally

Rosalind Benedet, N.P.

This unique book helps a woman through the journey of breast cancer once she has undergone surgery. Ms. Benedet, an oncology nurse, covers such topics as recovery at home, coping emotionally, body image, choosing a prosthesis, reconstructive surgery, nutrition, exercise, preventing lymphedema, and follow-up treatment, including chemotherapy and radiation. 170 pages

$14.95

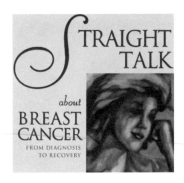

Straight Talk About Breast Cancer: From Diagnosis to Recovery

Suzanne Braddock, M.D., John Edney, M.D., Jane Kercher, M.D., Melanie Morrissey Clark

After recovering from a double mastectomy and chemotherapy, Suzanne Braddock, M.D. wanted to write a book that answers the pressing questions women have after a diagnosis. She achieved that goal with this book, which is now used by hospitals, clinics, and state health departments across the country. Eight pages of reconstruction photos. 172 pages

$14.95

Consumer Health Titles from Addicus Books
Visit our online catalog at www.AddicusBooks.com

After Mastectomy—Healing Physically and Emotionally · · · · · · · · · · · · · $14.95
Cancers of the Mouth and Throat—A Patient's Guide to Treatment · · · · · · · · · $14.95
Cataracts: A Patient's Guide to Treatment · · · · · · · · · · · · · · · · · · · $14.95
Colon & Rectal Cancer—A Patient's Guide to Treatment · · · · · · · · · · · · · $14.95
Coping with Psoriasis—A Patient's Guide to Treatment · · · · · · · · · · · · · $14.95
Coronary Heart Disease—A Guide to Diagnosis and Treatment · · · · · · · · · · · $15.95
Exercising Through Your Pregnancy · $17.95
The Fertility Handbook—A Guide to Getting Pregnant · · · · · · · · · · · · · · $14.95
The Healing Touch—Keeping the Doctor/Patient
    Relationship Alive Under Managed Care · · · · · · · · · · · · · · · · · · · $9.95
LASIK—A Guide to Laser Vision Correction · · · · · · · · · · · · · · · · · · $14.95
Living with P.C.O.S.—Polycystic Ovarian Syndrome · · · · · · · · · · · · · · $14.95
Lung Cancer—A Guide to Treatment & Diagnosis · · · · · · · · · · · · · · · · $14.95
The Macular Degeneration Source Book · $14.95
The Non-Surgical Facelift Book—A Guide to Facial Rejuvenation Procedures · · · · $14.95
Overcoming Postpartum Depression and Anxiety · · · · · · · · · · · · · · · · · $14.95
A Patient's Guide to Dental Implants · $14.95
Prescription Drug Addiction—The Hidden Epidemic · · · · · · · · · · · · · · · $15.95
Prostate Cancer—A Patient's Guide to Treatment · · · · · · · · · · · · · · · · $14.95
Simple Changes: The Boomer's Guide to a Healthier, Happier Life · · · · · · · · · $9.95
A Simple Guide to Thyroid Disorders · $14.95
Straight Talk About Breast Cancer From Diagnosis to Recovery · · · · · · · · · · $14.95
The Stroke Recovery Book—A Guide for Patients and Families · · · · · · · · · · · $14.95
The Surgery Handbook—A Guide to Understanding Your Operation · · · · · · · · · $14.95
Understanding Lumpectomy—A Treatment Guide for Breast Cancer · · · · · · · · · $14.95
Understanding Parkinson's Disease—A Self-Help Guide · · · · · · · · · · · · · · $14.95

Organizations, associations, corporations, hospitals, and other groups may qualify for special discounts when ordering more than 24 copies. For more information, please contact the Special Sales Department at Addicus Books. Phone (402) 330-7493.

Email: info@AddicusBooks.com

Please send:

_____copies of_____

(Title of book)

at $_____each   TOTAL   _____

Nebr. residents add 5.5% sales tax   _____

Shipping/Handling
  $4.00 for first book.
  $1.00 for each additional book.   _____

TOTAL ENCLOSED: _____

Name _____

Address _____

City_____State_____Zip _____

☐   Visa   ☐   Master Card   ☐   Am. Express

Credit card number _____Expiration date _____

Order by credit card, personal check or money order. Send to:

Addicus Books
Mail Order Dept.
P.O. Box 45327
Omaha, NE 68145
Or, order TOLL FREE: **800-352-2873**